Socio-Cultural Insights of Childbirth in South Asia

This book analyses the significant socio-cultural factors impacting childbirth experiences of women living in remote and complex social settings.

This book challenges the notion that childbirth is a universal biological event which women experience in their reproductive lives and provides an in-depth social perspective of understanding childbirth. Drawing on evocative stories of women living in the Himalayas, the author discusses how childbirth should be supported to enable women to take control and ownership of their experiences. Based on extensive research undertaken in remote mountain regions of Nepal, this book provides evidence for and discussion of childbirth in the context of other countries, cultures and communities. Utilising a feminist perspective, this book critiques medical control of childbirth and argues in favour of giving power to women so that they can make decisions which are right for them. In doing so, the author unpacks complexities associated with women's lives in remote communities and highlights the significance of addressing broader determinants impacting birth outcomes and valuing childbirth traditions to ensure cultural safety for women, families and societies.

Through exploring the wide range of factors influencing women and their childbirth experiences, this book offers a new model for childbirth that policymakers, practitioners, communities, educators, researchers and other professionals can use to make childbirth an empowering experience for women. It will be of interest to academics and professionals in the fields of public health, midwifery, health promotion, sociology and South Asian Studies.

Sabitra Kaphle is Lecturer of Public Health at Central Queensland University, Australia. Her research focuses on health and social issues in South Asia and sub-Saharan countries.

Routledge Contemporary South Asia Series

Bangladesh and International Law
Edited by Mohammad Shahabuddin

Terrorism and the US Drone Attacks in Pakistan
Killing First
Imdad Ullah

The Bangladesh Garment Industry and the Global Supply Chain
Choices and Constraints of Management
Shahidur Rahman

Globalising Everyday Consumption in India
History and Ethnography
Edited by Bhaswati Bhattacharya and Henrike Donner

Islam and Religious Change in Pakistan
Sufis and Ulema in 20th Century South Asia
Saadia Sumbal

Socio-Cultural Insights of Childbirth in South Asia
Stories of Women in the Himalayas
Sabitra Kaphle

The Geopolitics of Energy in South Asia
Energy Security of Bangladesh
Chowdhury Ishrak Ahmed Siddiky

Transdisciplinary Ethnography in India
Women in the Field
Edited by Rosa Maria Perez and Lina Fruzzetti

Socio-Cultural Insights of Childbirth in South Asia

Stories of Women in the Himalayas

Sabitra Kaphle

Routledge
Taylor & Francis Group

LONDON AND NEW YORK

First published 2022
by Routledge
2 Park Square, Milton Park, Abingdon, Oxon OX14 4RN

and by Routledge
605 Third Avenue, New York, NY 10158

Routledge is an imprint of the Taylor & Francis Group, an informa business

© 2022 Sabitra Kaphle

British Library Cataloguing-in-Publication Data
A catalogue record for this book is available from the British Library

Library of Congress Cataloging-in-Publication Data
A catalog record for this book has been requested

ISBN: 978-0-367-53804-0 (hbk)
ISBN: 978-0-367-54637-3 (pbk)
ISBN: 978-1-003-08994-0 (ebk)

Typeset in Times New Roman
by Apex CoVantage, LLC

This book is dedicated to my parents, who gave me life, and to my two daughters Sampada and Reva, who inspire me to live a meaningful life.

Contents

Illustrations

Figures

Table

Preface

On the afternoon of the 1 June 2019, I got a call from my sister to say our beloved mother had died. It would have soon been time to celebrate her 70th birthday, and I was in shock for 24 hours. Her death was sudden, and I was half a world away and unable to make the funeral. I lived in tears for months and found it hard to accept her loss.

Of Mum's four children, I was the only one that she gave birth to in hospital. It was not the practice, but with me she had no choice. She had gone through three days of severe bleeding in the village, and I was not yet due to be born. My dad came home for the weekend and found my mum fighting for two lives – her own and mine. He took her to the hospital, which was 40 km away. The hope was to save the life of my mother, so she could look after the three young children remaining at home.

Thank you to the midwives who worked hard to save the lives of both of us. I was born premature with little hope of survival, and I feel incredibly lucky to have spent my first 15 years of life in the village. Unfortunately, there are many mothers and babies around the world still fighting for their lives every day. I am writing this book to shine some light on these circumstances and to try to enhance their chances of survival.

There was a dark room without a window in the corner of our village house where my mother gave birth to her other three children. After 17 years, my sister-in-law came back from the capital city to give birth to her second baby in that same corner of the house. My mum supported the birth, and a healthy baby girl was born. I was curious to understand why my sister-in-law decided to come to the village to give birth. This prompted me to learn more about the social and cultural significance of birth experiences.

My grandmother died five years ago at the age of 101 and was my main source of knowledge to learn the traditions and culture of childbirth. She gave birth each time in the Goth (animal shed) and experienced several losses along the way. She supported the births of all my aunties and my mum in the village. One of my aunties got pregnant 19 times but none of the babies survived, and she died in her forties. Listening to the childbirth stories of my grandmother, my aunties, my mother and observing my sister-in-law confined to a dark room for childbirth and the subsequent 21 days – encouraged me to become a midwife.

I still remember how we were rushed to the library to get hold of limited copies of "Myles Textbook for Midwives" on the first day of the midwifery course. After saving some snack money, I managed to purchase a copy of the book to read during the holidays in my village. When I started reading the book to learn the procedures, I prepared myself to be an efficient midwife and apply that knowledge during clinical placement. However, I felt uncomfortable about the way we were treating women giving birth in hospital. They were confined to the "delivery bed" with stirrups on their legs and were forced to follow instructions. At this moment, I saw women as machines, while we were the operators. There was no choice or options open to these women for discussion; they were not even allowed to ask questions. The power rested with the doctors and midwives; women were voiceless. I wanted to quit halfway through the course, but my family insisted that I complete it. Despite the workload, I tried to spend more time with women. This enabled me to understand why my sister-in-law decided to give birth in the village.

I knew from the beginning that a clinical role was not for me. I could not accept the culture of denying a voice and choice to those coming to the hospital. The relationships between providers and recipients were mechanical. I left the hospital job and decided to work in the community. I took a role that involved supporting women in rural villages to empower themselves. I had to walk for days to spend time with rural women who gathered at night, so they could learn to read and write. Their commitment to attending night classes was phenomenal. One day a woman burst into tears sharing her feelings about being able to read a letter sent by her husband working overseas. I was happy being able to make a difference in their lives. I listened to them, I valued their interests and worked with them to find solutions. In this way, I gained trust from these women and villagers to allow me to help them to live in the way they wanted. This experience empowered me to focus on a community-based model of care.

After two years of working with groups of underprivileged women in rural villages, I had to leave community work. My family wanted me to sit the public service exam, which I felt I had to do. After that, I got an offer of work in a regional hospital, which I felt duty bound to accept, so I started working as a midwife on a busy ward.

There were only two midwives rostered for the night shift, and we would usually have 10-12 women giving birth. It was never easy, but it felt rewarding to see mothers happy with their newly born babies. I was glad to be able to listen to and give support to women. However, not every shift ended with celebration. Sometimes mothers did not win their battles for life. And sometimes they survived but not their babies. The survival of mothers and babies was far from guaranteed with the available medical care. All too often, it was not entirely clear why either mother or baby had died, and this upset me.

One day a friend of mine was expecting twins and was brought to hospital urgently. Her brother called me in a panic as I was not around. I rushed to the hospital, organised blood supplies, spoke with the obstetric surgeon, comforted the families and sent her off to the theatre for an emergency caesarean. I looked around to find that her brother and husband were silent, emotionally restless and stressed. They were begging me for her survival. Her situation was complex. It took three hours to complete the surgery – luckily both my friend and her twins were alive. I was on the night shift that day. At around midnight, I went to see my friend and noticed something was not right. Her pulse was low, her blood pressure was down, her face was pale and movements were weak.

I called the surgeon urgently, and we had to take her back to the theatre. Her situation was critical with internal bleeding. The theatre team strived successfully to save her life, and after six hours she was out of danger and sharing a happy reunion with her twins and families. It was clear to me that if she were not my friend, that woman would not have been alive. Personally, I did not feel right about that as I wanted all women to get equal access to care, support and resources. We were a long way away from that.

In 2003, I decided to switch my profession to public health and came to Australia to get a postgraduate degree in primary health care. It was a totally different experience for me, the approach to teaching, the lifestyle and the social system. What I found was the same were inequities in health care – in particular, the gap between Indigenous and non-Indigenous Australians.

A year later, I got pregnant. Even though I was already an experienced midwife; I felt helpless in that situation. I missed the care, advice and attention of my mother. Compared to Nepal, the healthcare system in Australia was excellent but I felt the lack of emotional support. I lacked confidence in giving birth in Australia, so I went back home to have my first baby even though Nepal was going through one of its frequent periods of civil unrest and there was a curfew every day. For the last eight weeks of my pregnancy, I stayed with my mother-in-law in a small town in Nepal. I was still expected to follow the social norms, values and practices, and I did so. I started seeing the obstetrician at a local hospital to continue care.

When I knew my first daughter was coming, I was sitting on the floor after a long day working to prepare for a family event the next day, I felt some discomfort. We were already restricted to the house on account of a curfew, and my husband was staying in Kathmandu for his job (about a day's travel on public transport). As a first-time mother, I did not know exactly what was going to happen and what to expect overnight, so initially I decided not to tell anyone. The night started to become real when I felt the pain and some signs of labour. Around midnight, my mother-in-law noticed that I had been ducking in and out of the room. There was no prospect of an ambulance coming until the next morning, and I thought I was going to die as the pain grew and the hours dragged on without my husband and mother for support.

Somehow, I got through that night and was taken to the local hospital the next morning. Luckily enough, a friend of mine whom I studied nursing was on duty that morning. As soon as I saw her, all the pain, discomfort, stress and fear melted away; I felt sure that she would not let me die. This experience taught me the importance of being around people that you trust with your safety during childbirth. On that morning of 9 September, I experienced a normal birth and welcomed a healthy baby girl.

The hospital was overcrowded, and I was asked to rest on the dirty floor on a bare mattress after the birth. I did not feel safe in that environment. I asked the nurse to let me go home, but she refused, I was shattered. Under their rules, I needed to stay there for 24 hours to watch for bleeding and other complications. I spoke with the attending obstetrician and convinced him that I would feel better at home. Finally, he discharged me on the condition that I would be responsible for any problems arising after leaving the hospital. I agreed with their terms and went home feeling relieved but threatened by the system in the hospital.

I followed the tradition and secluded myself in a room with the baby without touching anything outside it or anybody for 11 days. Hindu mythology considers the period after birth a "polluted" time and forces women to isolate themselves with their newborn in a separate space – limiting movement, contact with people and everyday activities. I had no choice, so I listened to my mother-in-law for advice as she was the closest person to me. I felt emotionally safe but also vulnerable at the same time. This experience gave me deeper insight into what is important for women while giving birth and what they need to feel safe afterwards. It was not about medicine or hospital procedures for me – it was all about the people around me and the sense of comfort I gained from them.

After a month, I went to stay with my mum. It was the most significant moment of my life. Being the youngest in the family, I had never felt any responsibilities up until I had my first daughter. Being with my mum gave me a sense of confidence. I never had to worry about the baby, I just followed my mum's lead. When I moved to Kathmandu to stay with my husband, I was with the baby all the time. Life was busy but I started feeling a sense of isolation. Apart from the baby and myself, I had no idea what was happening in the outside world. There was no internet and no phone access at that time, and I was cut off from my friends in Australia. I knew that I needed to change the situation. One morning, I decided I would look for a job. I spoke with a friend who was teaching in a nursing college, and she confirmed that they needed a lecturer to start immediately. I went for an interview and got the job. Now the problem was how to manage this with a young baby given we had no family nearby. We found a childcare centre, and I started teaching the nursing and midwifery course. The new routine of motherhood and a fulltime job kept me going. It was an empowering experience to teach the social model of midwifery, so students could listen and respond to the needs of birthing women.

Although I was busy juggling life and work, I was interested in doing something more challenging and interesting. I applied for a job with UNICEF that involved two major tasks – establishing birthing centres to provide round-the-clock childbirth services and strengthening emergency obstetric care services in hospitals in rural and remote parts of Nepal. At the time, I had an 18-month-old baby (still breast fed) and my husband was about to leave to study in Europe. The role with UNICEF involved working in the most remote region in Nepal. As much as I wanted to take up the challenge and explore the remote mountains of Nepal, I had no one to support me with the baby. I had never travelled to that region of the country before and had no family or friends to ask for help.

But having been offered the job, I decided to take a risk and accept it. My mother-in-law took the baby from me the day before I planned to leave Kathmandu to travel to the regional town. I was confused about the decision and devastated to be separated from my baby. I could not think straight or live normally, and I knew deep down that I needed my baby with me.

I started a new job in a regional office. For the first five weeks, it was traumatic for me to live without my baby. Having rented a house, organised furniture and basic essentials, I decided to go and get my daughter and bring her back with me. As soon as I made the decision, an indefinite strike started in Nepal and I was confined to the house for 19 days, unable to return to home. I was in a new place, a new job and a new neighbourhood, and my baby was far away while I was trapped in the lockdown.

After the lockdown ended, I picked up my daughter and we began our lives together again. I had to struggle to find a babysitter at the start, but I was happy to be with her outside work hours. We had mother-daughter time back again. For short field trips, I used to leave her with the babysitter. When I had a long field trip, I started taking her and the babysitter with me. It was a very different life compared to now, but that experience was rewarding and made both of us more resilient. We learnt to live life in hardship and with challenges, just like many mothers and children in the remote areas we visited were experiencing.

I got to know many midwives, mothers and families living in remote areas. Life was not easy for them. In the village, the model of care during pregnancy and childbirth was women oriented. At the same time, we had to train these nurses and midwives to become skilled birth attendants (SBAs). The SBA model was medically oriented to save maternal and newborn lives and the challenge was to blend the two models.

We built many birthing centres, extended hospital services, delivered training, bought many items of advanced equipment and set up blood transfusion and caesarean section facilities where possible. But women were still not coming to the birthing centre or the hospital to give birth. Most of those physical resources – the hospital buildings and the equipment – made no difference to practices in the villages. I heard several stories of the deaths of mothers and babies and witnessed a few too. I knew this model of service was not working for women in remote areas. I decided to quit the job and start a PhD to understand factors influencing the pregnancy and childbirth experiences of women in remote mountain areas of Nepal. This decision brought me back to Australia to begin a new journey. Doing a PhD was a passion for me; it took me back to remote villages to gather the childbirth stories of women, and it was a purely authentic experience. It enabled me to learn more and to argue confidently.

Once I returned from Nepal and started pulling together the stories of women from the mountains, I got pregnant. It was about the right time to have a second child but not the perfect time with academic pressures. The first four months were hard, as I still had to teach part-time, write my PhD thesis, manage a six-year-old and go through horrible morning sickness. But by that time, I felt fortunate to be in a place where all services were available to me at my doorstep. Compared to those women in the mountains who shared their stories with me, I was highly privileged. I was diagnosed with gestational diabetes and had to go through all the routine clinical tests, diets and so on. I wanted to avoid those clinical routines and enjoy the pregnancy, but I was worried about the safety of my unborn child. I followed the guidelines and all the routines. I felt totally healthy. They referred me to the obstetric clinic from the midwife-led care just because I had gestational diabetes. I was not convinced by the decision they made but I had no choice. I went to the obstetric clinic and they planned for an elective caesarean even though there was nothing wrong with the baby or me. I wanted to have a normal birth, and I was confident that I could do it. I spoke with my midwife and insisted that I stay in her care. I decided not to go back to the obstetric clinic – I took that risk. She listened to me and respected my decision.

On the afternoon of 19 November 2011, after five hours of pain I gave birth to a healthy baby with the support of my midwife within 10 minutes of reaching the emergency department. Everything went well. In both instances of childbirth, I had to challenge medical notions of risk and go with my own decisions in order to experience what safety means to me. Fortunately, that worked well, but not all women are able to make decisions about how they want to experience childbirth and their decisions are not always supported. My own experiences, and the childbirth stories of other women that I have been privileged to hear, convinced me to write this book. I am hoping that this book will give inspiration to those who want to challenge the medical model and embrace the way they want to experience childbirth.

Now I have settled in Australia, my daughters are nine and 16 years old. I thought this was the time to share the stories of the women who trusted me. So, I started writing this book just after the world was hit by COVID-19. We are locked inside the house; I can sense the social and psychological impacts among women who are new mothers or are expecting to give birth in these circumstances. The matter is critical but there has been little attention or discussion paid to it. All the measures that have been put in place are to reduce transmission of the virus for the physical safety of populations – emotional well-being is hardly spoken about.

After I submitted the full manuscript of this book to Routledge I planned to go and visit my dad to surprise him and let him know I had published a book. It was my sense of giving back, I also wanted to go back to the village and talk with the students at the high school where I spent my schooling years. Instead my dad surprised me by leaving us suddenly with cardiac arrest on 26 February 2021. I felt devastated with the news as my dreams were shattered and I found myself lost. I realised that the whole life I lived up until now has meaning and the reason behind this were my parents. Comprehending the loss of both parents gives me pain, suffering and discomfort but their faith in me consistently reminds me of the purpose of my life and the passion to give voices to those who are powerless, marginalised and underprivileged. Though my parents aren't here to witness the change that I contribute to make a better community, I feel proud to live with the inspiration and legacy of giving back to those who are in need to entertain same opportunities as everyone else in the society.

Given what we have been through most recently due to the global pandemic, witnessed the impacts on vulnerable populations and learnt so far, I hope the world wakes up one day and our health system starts to look at things differently, so that everyone can experience better care and enjoy a better life. No matter where or how we are born – everyone should have a chance for survival. I want to be there to witness such change and to share this story with my daughters.

Acknowledgements

This book would not have been possible without the support of my long-time friends Heidi Cornelsen, Lareen Newman, La Vonne Jose, Louise Townend, Norm Jose and Ruth Campbell in Adelaide where I spent five years of my university life at Flinders University. Not only do I call Adelaide my first home in Australia but I also consider these friends my Australian family. Those weekend drives, Saturday gatherings and special parties you let me be part of made my life in a new country comforting and worthwhile. Driving back from Adelaide to Melbourne after Christmas 2019, a thought echoed in my mind about the doctoral thesis I had written: "this is such an important story to share." Thanks to all of you for your encouragement from day one of my life at Flinders University until the present moment. Without your genuine friendship, continuing support and trust this book would not have come to completion.

This book contains the stories of women who struggle to live every day in difficult social circumstances. My sincere thanks to all the women, their family members and other people from these remote mountain communities for their trust, authenticity and openness in sharing their stories as they were. Without these stories you shared with me, my dream of writing a book would not have been realised. I feel fortunate to have had the opportunity of listening to and sharing your stories.

Special thanks to these friends in Melbourne for agreeing to read initial drafts and helping me to bring them to the next level: Anita Trezona, Anna Kortschak, Francesca Coles, Jenny Kelly, Matt Surawski and Rick Wallace. I am grateful to you and your families for allowing you the time to go through the writing of a friend who grew up in a rural village in Nepal, went to a public school and learnt to write in English only when she first came to Australia to do a postgraduate degree in 2003 and yet committed to writing this book for publication. Your support has given me greater confidence in my ability to write in a language I did not grow up with and reach wider audiences.

To my friends, colleagues and supervisors, who supported me throughout the PhD and writing of this book – trusting I had original and valuable contributions to make – heartfelt thanks for your belief in me.

Thanks to Dorothea Schaefter and Alexandra de Brauw, the editorial team at Routledge – Taylor & Francis Group for your tremendous support along the way to getting this book published. Despite the chaos of 2020, you were always there to answer multiple questions and check if I need additional support.

Finally, thanks to my family for their love, support and care.

While preparing this book for publication, I was still grieving the loss of my own mother and having her in mind while writing helped sustain me. My mother-in-law was another courageous woman with whom I had the privilege of spending parts of my life. Although neither are still with me, I hope they hear my whisper of gratitude: "thank you for allowing me to learn about your life." My father – I lost suddenly at the final stage of getting this book published – always taught me to never give up my passions in life and encouraged me to work hard and cherish my dreams. My husband who I like to call as long-time friend Dr Rajan Kadel has always helped me to realise my dreams. My two daughters Sampada and Reva – I would like to thank them for their understanding and patience in coping with my busy schedule and accepting my promise to watch Netflix with them once this book is published.

To my 92-year-old grandfather who still worries about the success of his grand-children and expects me to become an influential person in creating positive social change, I thank you for leading the way and giving me the courage to do so. My sisters, brothers, aunts, uncles, nieces, nephews and other families, I am always thankful to you.

Thank you all for helping me to share these words with you. Enjoy reading them. Namaste!

Outline of the book

Chapter 1. Introduction: socio-cultural insights into childbirth in South Asia

This chapter provides a basis for understanding the socio-cultural perspective by introducing evidence, concepts and reasoning for taking this approach to make meaning of childbirth experiences of women. It starts by discussing the differences in how childbirth is viewed in medical and social literature. This is followed by a brief discussion around the social view of childbirth including concepts of risk, choice, trust and safety. It provides the arguments to give women authority and power to decide where and how the birth should occur and sets the logic behind using childbirth stories of women from remote mountains of Nepal to set a strong agenda to take the socio-cultural context of childbirth into the account for policy and practice.

Chapter 2. Socio-cultural perspective of childbirth

This chapter explores the underpinning philosophies behind the socio-cultural perspective of childbirth drawing evidence from wide ranges of literature and theories. It highlights the significance of giving women power and authority to control the birthing process to make women feel empowered within their socio-cultural setting where birth occurs. It begins by explaining the significance and relevance of the social model of childbirth for women in cross-cultural settings. It argues that childbirth has significant social and cultural meaning in both non-Western and Western communities. It provides a critical discussion on various dimensions of the socio-cultural perspective and draws on the concept of oppression to liberation and argues to make childbirth an empowering experience to all women.

Chapter 3. Childbirth research in complex social settings: methodological reflections

This chapter explores various methodological complexities that researchers experience and offers possible strategies to manage the research process in an ethical, respectful and standard way. Drawing on the author's experiences, it argues for the significance of acknowledging the context of participants from socially vulnerable and culturally unique communities for research as a rewarding and empowering experience. It acknowledges that conducting research in a complex social setting involves managing challenging ethical, moral and methodological complexities and highlights the vital importance that researchers first understand the social context of participants, respect their status and take a flexible approach to adapt cultural needs, personal preferences, unexpected situations and social-familial expectations.

Chapter 4. Tradition, culture and spirituality: God inside

This chapter provides significant insights on women's trust to culture, tradition, spirituality, belief system, local knowledge and social norms to create a sense of childbirth-related safety. Drawing on experiences of women in remote mountain areas in Nepal, it confirms that the underpinning socio-cultural constructs and practices shape their childbirth. The lived experiences of women substantiate that when women can give birth within their community setting, their perception of childbirth safety is more likely to enhance as they feel threatened in an institutional environment. This has resulted in increased conformity to continue childbirth tradition and cultural practice for remote mountain women. Childbirth stories that women shared provide significant socio-cultural insights to improve maternal and newborn health outcomes in socially complex communities.

Chapter 5. Women, family members and significant others: paradox of power

This chapter draws the multiplicity of relationships that remote mountain women related to had paradoxical power interactions which led to complexities, contradictions and negotiations in constructing collective birthing experiences. It confirms that the patterns of social relations are influenced by ideological and material conditions of gender, knowledge, status quo and social position. Furthermore, it examines the context of socio-political processes that shape the healthcare system to operate against the choices and preferences of women, making services inaccessible in cultural, physical and social terms resulting in women's reluctance to seek the medical help with higher reliance on traditional knowledge and support available in the community.

Chapter 6. A complex array of factors: too far and too hard

This chapter focuses on wide ranges of cultural, social, structural and political determinants, which are critical to childbirth experiences of women and are beyond the capacity of the medical model to address while aiming to improve maternal and newborn survival. Drawing on the scenario that women's everyday life circumstances play critical role in childbirth and often leave them without any access to basic services to stay healthy during pregnancy, childbirth and postnatal period, it urges policymakers and service providers to consider the impacts of broader determinants to provide culturally responsive, emotionally-physically safe and appropriate services to women. It argues that asking women to attend hospital to give birth is not a practical or realistic and justified solution to improve maternal and newborn survival in these remote villages and emphasise the need for context specific policy and programmes.

Chapter 7. Insights for policy and practice: the woman centred, culturally safe, empowering and collaborative (WCEC) model of childbirth

This chapter proposes a collaborative model to promote the active engagement of various sectors including community, family and women in designing and providing high-quality care to women. It outlines the relevance of a woman centred, culturally safe, empowering and collaborative (WCEC) model of childbirth to enable improved access, choices and appropriateness of services to all women in the community. The WCEC model provides a guiding framework for designing context-specific policies and services to promote the maternal, perinatal and newborn health outcomes across different settings. It argues that using a collaborative approach to make decisions around policies, resourcing and service design could create an enabling environment to address the existing inequalities in maternal and newborn health outcomes.

Chapter 8. Conclusion: possibilities for positive childbirth experiences

This chapter sums up the critical insights into understanding the context of childbirth in socially complex and vulnerable settings. It acknowledges that childbirth is a complex personal and social experience for many women. Based on the voices of women, family members, stakeholders, service providers and the community, it argues for a community-based collaborative approach to improve the survival of mothers and babies in remote communities of Nepal which could be tailored to similar social settings.

1 Introduction

Socio-cultural insights into childbirth in South Asia

Introduction

> Juna has not travelled outside her district in her entire life and she doesn't know her actual age. She referred to the year of a big earthquake to get a sense of her age. She gave herself the approximate age of 42 and she looked significantly older than her made up age. Juna was not even 10 when she got married and she would have been around 16 to experience her first pregnancy. The current pregnancy was her seventh pregnancy, and she lives about three hours walks from the district hospital. She gave birth to her previous six children at Goth (cow sheds) and followed 30 days birth pollution practice for spiritual reasons. She was glad that everything went well, and she did not have any bad fortune. This time she went to hospital for one check-up, a first-time experience. Juna did not feel right about going to hospital. She returned home and decided to give birth in the same Goth and continued the tradition in the same way she did for the past six births.

Childbirth as a social and cultural event has hardly been discussed in mainstream medical literature. Obstetricians, midwives, and other healthcare providers were pushed to work within the set frameworks, protocols and routine procedures, mostly in an institutional setting. Only after 1970 sociologists started to write in mainstream literature highlighting the cross-cultural significance of childbirth [1–6]. Oakley's publications "Becoming a Mother" and "Women Confined: Towards a Sociology of Childbirth" provided strong critiques of a medical and institutional model of interventions and offered a social framework of childbirth. The notion of risks, choice and safety in childbirth has been defined differently in medical and sociological literature, which is putting women in a complex space while making decisions around where to give birth, from whom to seek support and how they would like that experience to be. The medicalisation and use of technology in childbirth made women's experiences more mechanical which threatened their emotional safety. Nevertheless, it is important to acknowledge the efforts of both the medical and social models of childbirth in preventing related deaths, illness and problems [7].

Globally, approximately 295,000 women died due to pregnancy and childbirth-related causes in 2017, of which 94% of deaths occurred in low-resource settings.

Nearly one-fifth of these deaths were in South Asia [8]. Similarly, 2.5 million children died in the first month of life in 2018 and about the same number of babies were stillborn in 2015 [8]. Despite the effort made under the Millennium Development Goals (MDG) and Sustainable Development Goals (SDG), disparities in maternal, newborn and child health outcomes between developed and developing countries remain wide. While looking at these numbers and inequities, it is critical to examine why mothers are dying during childbirth and what could be done to prevent these deaths, especially in low resource settings.

There has been ongoing advocacy on utilising the social support for women during childbirth to minimise risks of dying [9–11]. Sadly, it has not yet been translated to change in the way maternity care is provided to women, which remains mostly medically driven. It still raises a serious question about the healthcare systems in most of the developing countries which have failed to ensure the survival of mothers and babies. This clearly signifies the role that social, cultural, economic and political factors play in designing and delivering care to women during pregnancy and childbirth.

Childbirth is a powerful personal event as well as a significant social experience for women of any society [12–14]. Despite the similar physiological process, women in different cultures and societies experience childbirth differently [15–27]. Therefore, understanding the childbirth experiences of women must entail understanding their culture, tradition, belief system and social values [28]. It has been argued consistently that the degree and type of women's choice and control depend on the construct of society where they experience childbirth [29–37]. Factors such as gender, power, social status, geography and the economy further impact women's choice and control about their childbirth. The influence of these factors, which are known as social determinants has been critical to reduce maternal and newborn mortality in developing countries.

In most parts of South Asia, childbirth is considered as a socially and culturally rich event with special traditions and rituals. Many women continue their traditional practices during pregnancy, childbirth and the postnatal period even when they migrate to other countries. Some strong belief and traditional practice restrict women from seeking medical care when needed, and this increases the risk of illness and deaths [38]. Common factors such as the concept of purity and pollution during and after childbirth, the use of traditional healers, construct of health and illness being related to deities, beliefs related to food, myths around what is accepted and now influence pregnancy and childbirth found to be critical to shape childbirth experiences [39]. In these societies, childbirth is considered as a natural process and the tendency to seek medical help only occurs when there are serious problems – which is normally the last option.

Although there is not enough evidence to confirm the correlation of the sociocultural factors to birth outcomes, limited research shows that South Asian born women are two times more likely to experience late pregnancy stillbirths than locally born women accessing the same public maternity services [40–42]. Nevertheless, consistent emphasis has been given to examine the influence of wider determinants to childbirth experiences of women to improve birth outcomes [43–45].

This book provides both social and cultural insights focusing on the wider determinants and practices related to childbirth in the context of South Asia. Drawing childbirth stories of women from the remote mountain villages of Nepal, I argue for a collaborative model of childbirth to promote maternal and newborn survival in cross-cultural settings.

Childbirth: medical or socio-cultural event

Public health research focuses on reducing inequalities of health outcomes related to childbirth within and between nations to prevent adverse results including the unnecessary deaths of mothers and babies in community settings [46–49]. In developing countries, there is significantly higher prevalence of childbirth-related complications leading to the deaths of mothers and newborn babies [50–54]. The South Asia region still has unacceptably high mortality and morbidity rates [55–60]. Childbirth is medically defined as a physiological phenomenon which denies the significance of maintaining social, cultural, spiritual and emotional safety for women. As a result, medical literature has heavy focus on physical risks and use of clinical measures and technologies to avert risks [26, 61–64].

Many sociologists challenged the way childbirth is viewed and managed medically as failing to acknowledge the influences of socio-cultural dimensions of women [64–68]. Medical understanding of childbirth does not acknowledge the traditional birthing practices which exist in many communities around the world; instead, women are blamed for not using the clinical services [69–73]. Public health researchers argue that childbirth outcomes are associated with social determinants rather than medical determinants because of the socio-cultural circumstances of women where they live and work [56, 74–85]. Thus, the experience that women develop during childbirth is impacted by the complex interactions of medical, social, cultural, political, spiritual and economic factors [80, 85–87]. In that lens, childbirth and its associated mortality rates amongst South Asian countries is a serious concern which needs attention of all sectors and services.

The socio-cultural perspective of childbirth emphasises the role of relationships and interactions within the particular social system. In that line, childbirth knowledge, beliefs and practices are shaped differently in diverse socio-cultural settings [88]. This is further highlighted by Baum [85], who takes the broader social view and urges us to analyse the influence of critical relationships including gender and power relations in determining health outcomes. This perspective is consistent with The Alma Ata [89, 90] and subsequent charters [91, 92] to consider social, political and structural determinants impacting health and well-being of populations.

Concept of socio-cultural in childbirth

The concept of socio-cultural in this book encompasses a range of dimensions: social relationships; cultural values, beliefs, traditions and practices; economic, political and structural factors; religion and spirituality; gender, caste and ethnicity; traditional knowledge; power dynamics; education; literacy and family and societal conditions. These dimensions are derived from social science litera-ture and I am using this term consistently to refer to either all or some of these dimensions of childbirth while analysing, understanding and describing women's experiences. I am taking a broader view to examine the influence of wide ranges of socio-cultural factors to childbirth experiences of women.

The socio-cultural view of childbirth emerged historically from the declaration of Alma Ata which recognises that achieving health requires action not only in health but also in many social, political and economic sectors [90]. Primary health care (PHC) draws attention to address basic social needs such as housing, afford-able food supplies and proper nutrition, adequate supply of safe water and basic sanitation, safety from violence and social support which are important to achieve better health. PHC has acknowledged the influence of broader social and environ-mental factors to achieve positive health outcomes [93] and pushed for increased community participation and utilisation of local resources while making health-related decisions [74, 94, 95]. The Ottawa Charter for Health Promotion [92] draws PHC principles and reaffirms that improvement in health requires better education, income, sustainable resources, social justice and equity. The Bang-kok Charter for Health Promotion added the spiritual dimension to health, sup-porting the broader socio-cultural perspective of health and well-being [91]. The 30th anniversary of the Declaration of Alma Ata provided a renewed approach to health by focusing on addressing social inequalities [89].

The Commissions on Social Determinants of Health provided a framework to address wide ranges of factors impacting health and well-being of popula-tions [81]. Labonte and colleagues [96–98] consistently reaffirm that action on social determinants requires focus on more research and changes in policy and practice. Social determinants framework has been used widely to address the broader social factors causing inequalities in maternal and newborn health out-comes [79, 99, 100]. The Countdown to 2015 Decade Report [8] emphasises that more work is needed to improve maternal, newborn and child survival. It has been argued that socio-cultural circumstances are often complex and require appropri-ate interventions for reduction of maternal, perinatal and newborn mortality [101]. In this environment, understanding the complexities in which childbirth occurs is pertinent to policy, practice and programme levels.

Concept of safety, choice, risk and trust in childbirth

The concepts of safety, choice, risk and trust form the basis of understanding childbirth experiences of women. These concepts are widely discussed in the lit-erature in relation to childbirth, but their meaning varies. There is a huge differ-ence in the way how these concepts are defined in the medical model and I intend to use these terms in this book as socially and culturally constructed concepts.

In socio-cultural perspective, the term safety signifies the influences of ranges of social and cultural factors in childbirth experiences [102–106]. In this sense, safety includes many components: a strong and supportive cultural belief system [16, 28, 104, 107–109]; the presence of tradition and spirituality [24, 63]; good and supportive relationships [110, 111]; trust and respect in relationships [112–114]; childbirth as an ordinary part of everyday life [3, 115]; birthing in traditional/community/home settings [31, 32, 116, 117]; the presence of family members at birth [118, 119]; spiritual beliefs and practices [22, 120]; women exercising some control in the childbirth process [121–124]; support of a trusted person during childbirth [118, 119]; freedom from risk and uncertainties of survival [108, 125–129]; and being able to exercise lay or traditional knowledge [128, 129]. The presence of one or more of these components signifies degrees of safety that women experience during childbirth and this is how the term safety is used in this book.

The concept of choice focuses on where and how women would like to experience birth. This notion of choice is influenced by various social and cultural factors and relates with the way safety is described and viewed by women [130–132]. The use of the term choice in this book refers to the opportunities and resources available to women to decide about childbirth in a way that is socially and culturally appropriate. In this context, choices made by women during childbirth are the outcome of the wider social values, relationship patterns, power influences, cultural beliefs and material circumstances which is supported by the theoretical construct of structure and agency. This notion of choice acknowledges the fact that decisions women have made are not based on their individual interest or preferences but informed by how social discourse and cultural construct operate to form knowledge about risk and safety.

The medical construction of risk generates concerns about the safety of women during childbirth [133], as the notion of risk in medicine focuses only on physical aspects of childbirth with scientific calculation of potential hazard without taking women's emotional well-being into account. Childbirth has been impacted hugely by risk technologies to shift attention away from the safety of mothers to the safety of the unborn baby in medical practice [112]. The social construction of risks critiques medical discourse, which describe risks in more technical and statistical fashions and involves any acts that threaten one or more aspects of safety during childbirth. This construction relies on risk perception, risk knowledge and risky practices associated with childbirth within the context of women [134]. Their sense of risks could be physical, spiritual or emotional to determine where and how to give birth including postpartum care. I will use both the medical and social construction of risk in this book to analyse childbirth experiences of women according to their socio-cultural circumstances.

Luhmann [135] frames the function of trust as the "reduction of complexity." In that context, trust occurs when a decision is made based on familiarity, expectation and risk knowledge which leads to the reduction of complexity and helps to develop a sense of safety [135]. Giddens's [126] concept of trust works well in circumstances of uncertainties and multiple choices where trust is linked to achieving an early sense of ontological security through screening potential threats or risks and danger. In this view, trust is basic to a "protective cocoon" which stands guard over the self in its dealings with everyday reality [136]. Giddens asserts that risk produced by modernisation and technology can be challenged by trust to create positive childbirth experiences [136]. Supporting Giddens's concept of "active trust," Banks and colleagues [112] acknowledge the importance of emergence of new social relations to facilitate a process of mutual narrative and emotional dis-closure. That mutual narrative in Giddens's view is not a priori predicated on class or social status but rather on the combination of choices that converge [112]. Both Luhmann [135] and Giddens [127] see trust as an effective tool for reducing the risk, complexities and uncertainties that exist in modern society. I use their notion of trust in this book as childbirth involves risks, uncertainties and complexities which could be managed effectively by establishing trust. The term trust in this book signifies a mutual relationship, reciprocal understanding and perceived ben-efits of action.

Theoretical concepts: social constructionism and critical feminism

I use social constructionism and critical feminism frameworks to understand the influences of various socio-cultural dimensions on childbirth experiences of women. This helps to give meaning and privilege to share their childbirth stories as an authentic source of knowledge.

The epistemological position of social constructionism implies that knowledge is the outcome of the interactions among individuals engaging in its construction. This approach informs an examination of how people make sense of their world, construct knowledge and respond to the same situation differently [137, 138]. How one person sees a phenomenon can be different to how another person inter-prets the same phenomenon [139, 140]. In this process, the meaning is dependent on the relationship between experiences and the concerned individual [141]. The relationship in this construction is guided by the social values of people and of those with which they interact [142]. The construction of childbirth knowledge is influenced by the socio-cultural values and the interactions between women, family members and other people involved. In this process, how one woman con-structs the meaning of their childbirth experiences can be different to how another woman constructs hers.

Lock and Strong [143] provide four key features of social constructionism. First, it is concerned with meaning and understanding with the focus on how knowledge is constructed. Second, meaning and understanding have their begin-ning in social interactions with shared agreement. Third, ways of meaning mak-ing, being inherently embedded in socio-cultural processes, are specific to times and places. Fourth, people are self-defining and socially constructed participants in their shared life. Social constructionism values the collective construction of childbirth knowledge and the influences of socio-cultural factors in the construc-tion of childbirth experiences. It sees childbirth knowledge as socially constructed experiences, which values the importance of interactions and relationships to give meaning to the experiences [144].

Critical feminism focuses on giving values to women's voices while exam-ining the influences of gendered ideology, power influences and social interac-tions on childbirth [111, 133]. It is a liberating approach which enables women to be part of a transformative process of enhancing safety during childbirth [145].

Critical feminism acknowledges that social change begins from everyday lives of women and attempts to minimise imposed hierarchies and exploitative relationships [146]. This approach encourages active involvement of women as research participants and considers women as an expert of their experiences [147]. Listening to childbirth stories of women enables us to understand the relationships and influences of socio-cultural factors validating the uniqueness of that experience.

Childbirth in the Himalayas: a unique collective experience

More than half (57%) of deaths among children under the age of five in South Asia occur in the first 28 days of life resulting in more than 1 million newborn deaths every year [148]. Out of the 2.6 million stillbirths occur every year globally, South Asia accounts for 37% [84]. National policies, reports, critique papers and research articles repeatedly report these numbers; mostly highlighting the challenge that South Asia still experiences in promoting maternal and newborn survival. Data support medical causes leading to higher maternal, perinatal, and newborn deaths in the region with some analyses of socio-economic disparities based on income quantile and geographic variations. Evidence lacks to examine the socio-cultural circumstances of childbirth in South Asia and does not acknowledge the role of collective social practice which is rich with traditions, rituals and culture in enhancing safety during childbirth.

All countries in South Asia have made significant investment towards the reduction of maternal, perinatal, newborn and child mortality and developed various innovative and targeted policies and strategies. Despite the national efforts, childbirth-related deaths are still higher among poor, vulnerable, disadvantaged, remote and rural populations. Evidence suggests that people living in the Himalayas have particularly poor social, economic and health status [149–152]. This is characterised by the higher fertility, morbidity and mortality rates existing in Nepal's remote mountain areas [149, 150, 153–155]. Murshed and Gates [156] suggest the difference in remote mountain areas is associated with limited access to basic resources and a strong preference of traditional healing systems. Other researchers further validated the difficulty of accessing medical services over traditional healing systems in the remote and rural areas of Nepal [7, 38, 149, 150, 154, 157, 158]. More than 90% of women living in the remote mountain areas of Nepal still give birth at home [154].

Childbirth experiences of rural Nepalese women are influenced by limited opportunities for choice [7, 38, 159–163]. In traditional gender roles, most women are considered inferior to men [164]. Even now, married women are expected to be at home and to serve their husband's family [165]. In this deeply rooted patriarchy, men are expected to take control of women and families. It has been evident in practice resulting in multiple pregnancies to satisfy husbands or other family members [166–169]. In this social system, the influence of the mother-in-law in women's childbirth experiences is critical [7, 38, 158, 170–172]. Although women of suburban and urban areas have shown success in empowering themselves in a variety of development sectors including health [152, 173–175], the situation for women living in remote mountain areas remains the same considering childbirth as an everyday chore in life [7, 38, 176].

A deeper understanding of childbirth practice in remote mountain areas is needed. The need for understanding the significance of socio-cultural factors related to childbirth has been highlighted by some researchers [158, 170, 177, 178]; however, little is known about women living in remote communities. With limited attempts to understand why women prefer giving birth at home and what factors influence their decisions, the health system tends to blame them for not accessing medical services [7, 158, 170, 179]. This is a critical question which I attempt to answer in this book using stories shared by women living remote mountain villages of Nepal, who sees childbirth as a collective social and cultural experiences. I conducted a research with women from remote mountain villages that aimed at understanding the factors influencing childbirth experiences. I also examined the relationships and impacts of various factors in childbirth. Using their stories, I will provide significant evidence to support the socio-cultural perspective of childbirth, which are applicable to any context of the society.

Conclusion

Pregnancy and childbirth have been defined as personal physiological experiences for women in the medical model. But for many women, giving birth is a socially, culturally and spiritually meaningful and collective experience. For women in South Asia, childbirth-related rituals, traditions, cultural practices and belief systems make this experience unique and overwhelming. The socio-cultural perspective allows to understand the complex nature of childbirth experiences within the context of women and helps to analyse the multiplicity of factors that are critical to make this experience safe and liberating to women.

In this context, the concept of risk and safety plays a significant role to determine the outcome of childbirth experiences. Taking critical feminist stand, arguments are made to give women authority and power to decide where and how the birth should occur by setting the logic behind to understand childbirth stories of women from remote mountains of Nepal, and by setting a strong agenda to take the socio-cultural context of childbirth into the account for service design, policy and practice in South Asia.

References

1   Oakley, A., *Trap of medicalised motherhood*. New Society, 1975. **34**(689): p. 639–645.
2   Oakley, A., *Wisewoman and medicine man: Changes in the management of childbirth*. The Rights and Wrongs of Women. 1976: p. 17–58.
3   Oakley, A., *Becoming a mother*. 1979: Schocken, New York.
4   Jordan, B., *Birth in four cultures: A cross-cultural investigation of childbirth in Yucatan, Holland, Sweden and the United States*. 1978: Eden, Montreal.
5   Jordan, B., *Birth in four cultures: A cross-cultural investigation of childbirth in Yucatan, Holland, Sweden, and the United States*. 1992: Waveland Press, Long Grove.

6   Kitzinger, S., *Ourselves as mothers: The universal experience of motherhood*. 1995: Addison Wesley Publishing Company, Boston.

7   Kaphle, S., H. Hancock, and L.A. Newman, *Childbirth traditions and cultural perceptions of safety in Nepal: Critical spaces to ensure the survival of mothers and newborn in remote mountain villages*. Midwifery, 2013. **29**(10): p. 1173–1181.

8   World Health Organisation, *Trends in maternal mortality 2000 to 2017: Estimates by WHO, UNICEF*. UNFPA, World Bank Group and the United Nations Population Division, Geneva. Retrieved April, 2019. **1**: p. 2020.

9   Sosa, R., et al., *The effect of a supportive companion on perinatal problems, length of labor, and mother-infant interaction*. New England Journal of Medicine, 1980. **303**(11): p. 597–600.

10   Oakley, A., *Social support and perinatal outcome*. International Journal of Technology Assessment in Health Care, 1985. **1**(4): p. 843–854.

11   Chalmers, I., M. Enkin, and M.J. Keirse, *Effective care in pregnancy and childbirth: Pregnancy*. 1989: Oxford University Press, New York.

12   Carpenter, M., *The birthing experience: Towards an ecosystem approach*. 2009: PhD Dissertation, University of South Africa, Pretoria, South Africa.

13   Lemay, C., *Reclaiming meanings for birth, pain and risk within the home setting*. Promoting Normal Birth: Research, Reflections and Guidelines. 2011: Fresh Heart Publishing, Durham.

14   Reynolds, J.L., *Post-traumatic stress disorder after childbirth: The phenomenon of traumatic birth*. CMAJ, 1997. **156**(6): p. 831–835.

15   Callister, L.C., *Making meaning: Women's birth narratives*. Journal of Obstetric, Gynaecologic, and Neonatal Nursing, 2004. **33**(4): p. 508–518.

16   Callister, L.C. and I. Khalaf, *Spirituality in childbearing women*. The Journal of Perinatal Education, 2010. **19**(2): p. 16–24.

17   Callister, L.C., S. Semenic, and J.C. Foster, *Cultural and spiritual meanings of childbirth: Orthodox Jewish and Mormon women*. Journal of Holistic Nursing, 1999. **17**(3): p. 280–295.

18   Callister, L.C., K. Vehvilainen-Julkunen, and S. Lauri, *Cultural perceptions of childbirth: A cross-cultural comparison of childbearing women*. Journal of Holistic Nursing, 1996. **14**(1): p. 66–78.

19   Khalaf, I.a. and L.C. Callister, *Cultural meanings of childbirth: Muslim women living in Jordan*. Journal of Holistic Nursing, 1997. **15**(4): p. 373–388.

20   Bharj, K. and M. Cooper, *The social context of childbirth and motherhood*. Myles' Textbook for Midwives. 2009: Elsevier Churchill Livingstone, Sydney.

21   Di Ciano, T., et al., *Postnatal social support group needs and explanatory models of Iraqi Arabic speaking women in the year following the birth of their baby in Perth, Western Australia*. Advances in Mental Health, 2010. **9**(2): p. 162–176.

22   Hall, J., *Spirituality and labour care*. Essential Midwifery Practice: Intrapartum Care. 2010: p. 235–251.

23   Benza, S. and P. Liamputtong, *Pregnancy, childbirth and motherhood: A meta-synthesis of the lived experiences of immigrant women*. Midwifery, 2014. **30**(6): p. 575–584.

24   Liamputtong, P., Pregnancy, childbirth and traditional beliefs and practices in Chiang Mai, Northern Thailand, in *Childbirth across Cultures*. 2009: Springer, New York. p. 175–184.

25   Rice, P.L. and J. Lumley, *Childbirth and soul loss: The case of a Hmong woman*. Medical Journal of Australia, 1994. **160**(9): p. 577–578.

26   Sawyer, A., et al., *Women's experiences of pregnancy, childbirth, and the postnatal period in the Gambia: A qualitative study.* British Journal of Health Psychology, 2011. **16**(3): p. 528–541.

27   Schneider, D.A., *Beyond the baby: Women's narratives of childbirth, change and power.* 2009: Smith College School for Social Work, Northampton.

28   Callister, L.C. and I. Khalaf, Culturally diverse women giving birth: Their stories, in *Childbirth across cultures.* 2009: Springer, New York. p. 33–39.

29   Dahlen, H.G., L.M. Barclay, and C.S. Homer, *Processing the first birth: Journeying into 'motherland'.* Journal of Clinical Nursing, 2010. **19**(13-14): p. 1977–1985.

30   Dahlen, H.G., L.M. Barclay, and C.S.E. Homer, *The novice birthing: Theorising first-time mothers' experiences of birth at home and in hospital in Australia.* Midwifery, 2010. **26**(1): p. 53–63.

31   Douglas, V.K., *Childbirth among the Canadian Inuit: A review of the clinical and cultural literature.* International Journal of Circumpolar Health, 2006. **65**(2): p. 117–132.

32   Douglas, V.K., *The Inuulitsivik maternities: Culturally appropriate midwifery and epistemological accommodation.* Nursing Inquiry, 2010. **17**(2): p. 111–117.

33   Douglas, V.K., *The Rankin Inlet Birthing Centre: Community midwifery in the Inuit context.* International Journal of Circumpolar Health, 2011. **70**(2): p. 178–185.

34   Lindgren, H. and K. Erlandsson, *Women's experiences of empowerment in a planned home birth: A Swedish population-based study.* Birth, 2010. **37**(4): p. 309–317.

35   Lindgren, H.E., et al., *Perceptions of risk and risk management among 735 women who opted for a home birth.* Midwifery, 2010. **26**(2): p. 163–172.

36   Namey, E.E. and A.D. Lyerly, *The meaning of "control" for childbearing women in the US.* Social Science and Medicine, 2010. **71**(4): p. 769–776.

37   Snowden, A., et al., *Concurrent analysis of choice and control in childbirth.* BMC Pregnancy and Childbirth, 2011. **11**(1): p. 40.

38   Kaphle, S., *Uncovering the covered: Pregnancy and childbirth experiences of women living in remote mountain areas of Nepal.* 2012: Flinders University, School of Medicine, Discipline of Public Health, Adelaide.

39   Rozario, S. and G. Samuel, *Daughters of Hariti: Childbirth and female healers in South and Southeast Asia.* 2003: Routledge, London.

40   Davies-Tuck, M.L., M.-A. Davey, and E.M. Wallace, *Maternal region of birth and stillbirth in Victoria, Australia 2000–2011: A retrospective cohort study of Victorian perinatal data.* PLoS One, 2017. **12**(6): p. e0178727.

41   Drysdale, H., et al., *Ethnicity and the risk of late-pregnancy stillbirth.* Medical Journal of Australia, 2012. **197**(5): p. 278–281.

42   Gardosi, J., et al., *Maternal and fetal risk factors for stillbirth: Population-based study.* BMJ, 2013. **346**.

43   Amjad, S., et al., *Social determinants of health and adverse maternal and birth outcomes in adolescent pregnancies: A systematic review and meta-analysis.* Paediatric and Perinatal Epidemiology, 2019. **33**(1): p. 88–99.

44   Giurgescu, C., *Social determinants of maternal health and birth outcomes.* The American Journal of Maternal and Child Nursing, 2017. **42**(1): p.7.

45   Gadson, A., E. Akpovi, and P.K. Mehta, Exploring the social determinants of racial/ethnic disparities in prenatal care utilization and maternal outcome, in *Seminars in Perinatology.* 2017: Elsevier, Amsterdam.

46   Luo, Z.-C., et al., *Birth outcomes in the Inuit-inhabited areas of Canada.* CMAJ, 2010. **182**(3): p. 235–242.

47   Judge, K., *Inequalities in infant mortality: Patterns, trends, policy responses and emerging issues in Canada, Chile, Sweden and the United Kingdom.* Health Sociology Review, 2009. **18**(1): p. 12–24.

48   Pattenden, S., et al., *Geographical variation in infant mortality, stillbirth and low birth weight in Northern Ireland, 1992–2002.* Journal of Epidemiology Community Health, 2011. **65**(12): p. 1159–1165.

49   Rosenthal, L. and M. Lobel, *Explaining racial disparities in adverse birth outcomes: Unique sources of stress for Black American women.* Social Science and Medicine, 2011. **72**(6): p. 977–983.

50   Beck, S., et al., *The worldwide incidence of preterm birth: A systematic review of maternal mortality and morbidity.* Bulletin of the World Health Organization, 2010. **88**: p. 31–38.

51   Carlo, W.A., et al., *High mortality rates for very low birth weight infants in developing countries despite training.* Paediatrics, 2010. **126**(5): p. e1072–e1080.

52   Carlo, W.A., et al., *Newborn-care training and perinatal mortality in developing countries.* New England Journal of Medicine, 2010. **362**(7): p. 614–623.

53   McClure, E.M., et al., *Stillbirth in developing countries: A review of causes, risk factors and prevention strategies.* The Journal of Maternal, Foetal and Neonatal Medicine, 2009. **22**(3): p. 183–190.

54   Pattinson, R., et al., *Perinatal mortality audit: Counting, accountability, and overcoming challenges in scaling up in low-and middle-income countries.* International Journal of Gynaecology and Obstetrics, 2009. **107**: p. S113–S122.

55   Black, R.E., et al., *Global, regional, and national causes of child mortality in 2008: A systematic analysis.* The Lancet, 2010. **375**(9730): p. 1969–1987.

56   Boerma, T., et al., *Countdown to 2030: Tracking progress towards universal coverage for reproductive, maternal, newborn, and child health.* The Lancet, 2018. **391**(10129): p. 1538–1548.

57   Cousens, S., et al., *National, regional, and worldwide estimates of stillbirth rates in 2009 with trends since 1995: A systematic analysis.* The Lancet, 2011. **377**(9774): p. 1319–1330.

58   Friberg, I.K., et al., *Comparing modelled predictions of neonatal mortality impacts using LiST with observed results of community-based intervention trials in South Asia.* International Journal of Epidemiology, 2010. **39**(1): p. i11–i20.

59   George, K., et al., *Perinatal outcomes in a South Asian setting with high rates of low birth weight.* BMC Pregnancy and Childbirth, 2009. **9**(1): p. 5.

60   Lumbiganon, P., et al., *Method of delivery and pregnancy outcomes in Asia: The WHO global survey on maternal and perinatal health 2007–08.* The Lancet, 2010. **375**(9713): p. 490–499.

61   Haines, H., et al., *Cross-cultural comparison of levels of childbirth-related fear in an Australian and Swedish sample.* Midwifery, 2011. **27**(4): p. 560–567.

62   Kringeland, T., A.K. Daltveit, and A. Møller, *How does preference for natural childbirth relate to the actual mode of delivery? A population-based cohort study from Norway.* Birth, 2010. **37**(1): p. 21–27.

63   Lori, J.R. and J.S. Boyle, *Cultural childbirth practices, beliefs, and traditions in post-conflict Liberia.* Health care for women international, 2011. **32**(6): p. 454–473.

64   McCourt, C., *Cosmologies, concepts and theories: Time and childbirth in cross-cultural perspective.* 2009: Berghahn Books, Oxford.

65   Benoit, C., et al., *Medical dominance and neoliberalisation in maternal care provision: The evidence from Canada and Australia.* Social Science and Medicine, 2010. **71**(3): p. 475–481.

66   Harris, A., et al., *Challenges to maternal health care utilization among ethnic minority women in a resource-poor region of Sichuan Province, China.* Health Policy and Planning, 2010. **25**(4): p. 311–318.

67   Titaley, C.R., et al., *Why do some women still prefer traditional birth attendants and home delivery? A qualitative study on delivery care services in West Java Province, Indonesia.* BMC Pregnancy and Childbirth, 2010. **10**(1): p. 43.

68   Titaley, C.R., et al., *Why don't some women attend antenatal and postnatal care services? A qualitative study of community members' perspectives in Garut, Sukabumi and Ciamis districts of West Java Province, Indonesia.* BMC Pregnancy and Childbirth, 2010. **10**(1): p. 61.

69   Afsana, K. and S.F. Rashid, Constructions of birth in Bangladesh, in *Childbirth across cultures.* 2009: Springer. p. 123–135.

70   Goodburn, E.A., R. Gazi, and M. Chowdhury, *Beliefs and practices regarding delivery and postpartum maternal morbidity in rural Bangladesh.* Studies in Family Planning, 1995: p. 22–32.

71   Jeffery, P. and R. Jeffery, *Only when the boat has started sinking: A maternal death in rural north India.* Social Science and Medicine, 2010. **71**(10): p. 1711–1718.

72   Lang, J.B. and E.D. Elkin, *A study of the beliefs and birthing practices of traditional midwives in rural Guatemala.* Journal of Nurse-Midwifery, 1997. **42**(1): p. 25–31.

73   Moore, B., B. Alex-Hart, and I. George, *Utilization of health care services by pregnant mothers during delivery: A community based study in Nigeria.* East African Journal of Public Health, 2011. **8**(1): p. 48–50.

74   Freeman, T., et al., *Reaching those with the greatest need: How Australian primary health care service managers, practitioners and funders understand and respond to health inequity.* Australian Journal of Primary Health, 2011. **17**(4): p. 355–361.

75   Bhutta, Z.A., et al., *Countdown to 2015 decade report (2000–10): Taking stock of maternal, newborn, and child survival.* The Lancet, 2010. **375**(9730): p. 2032–2044.

76   Bhutta, Z.A., et al., *Maternal and child health: Is South Asia ready for change?* BMJ, 2004. **328**(7443): p. 816–819.

77   Brown, S. and J. Lumley, *Changing childbirth: Lessons from an Australian survey of 1336 women.* BJOG: An International Journal of Obstetrics and Gynaecology, 1998. **105**(2): p. 143–155.

78   Brown, S.J., et al., *Stressful life events, social health issues and low birthweight in an Australian population-based birth cohort: Challenges and opportunities in antenatal care.* BMC Public Health, 2011. **11**(1): p. 196.

79   Friel, S. and M.G. Marmot, *Action on the social determinants of health and health inequities goes global.* Annual Review of Public Health, 2011. **32**: p. 225–236.

80   Marmot, M., *Social determinants of health inequalities.* The Lancet, 2005. **365**(9464): p. 1099–1104.

81   Marmot, M., et al., *Closing the gap in a generation: Health equity through action on the social determinants of health.* The Lancet, 2008. **372**(9650): p. 1661–1669.

82   Houweling, T., A. Costello, and D. Osrin, Improving maternal and newborn survival through community intervention, in *The Routledge international handbook on global public health.* 2010: Routledge, London.

83   Houweling, T.A., et al., *Reaching the poor with health interventions: Programme-incidence analysis of seven randomised trials of women's groups to reduce newborn mortality in Asia and Africa.* Journal of Epidemiology Community Health, 2016. **70**(1): p. 31–41.

84 Lawn, J., *Maternal and child health – now, then, or when?* The Lancet, 2010. **375**(9730): p. 1957–1958.

85 Baum, F., *The new public health.* 2016: Oxford University Press, Oxford.

86 Kass, J.D., et al., *Health outcomes and a new index of spiritual experience.* Journal for the Scientific Study of Religion, 1991: p. 203–211.

87 Stainton Rogers, W., *Explaining health and illness: An exploration of diversity.* 1991: Harvester Wheatsheaf, London.

88 Teman, E., *Childbirth, midwifery and concepts of time – Edited by Christine McCourt; foreword: Ronnie Frankenberg.* Journal of the Royal Anthropological Institute, 2011. **17**(1): p. 196–197.

89 World Health Organisation, *Primary health care: Now more than ever.* 2008: World Health Organisation, Geneva.

90 World Health Organization, *Declaration of Alma-Ata international conference on primary health care held in Alma-Ata, USSR, 6–12 September.* 1978: World Health Organisation, Geneva.

91 World Health Organisation, *The Bangkok charter for health promotion in a globalised world.* 2005: World Health Organisation, Geneva.

92 World Health Organisation, *Ottawa charter for health promotion.* Health Promotion. 1986: World Health Organisation, Geneva.

93 Keleher, H., *Why primary health care offers a more comprehensive approach to tackling health inequities than primary care.* Australian Journal of Primary Health, 2001. **7**(2): p. 57–61.

94 Rifkin, S.B. and G. Walt, *Why health improves: Defining the issues concerning 'comprehensive primary health care' and 'selective primary health care'.* Social Science and Medicine, 1986. **23**(6): p. 559–566.

95 Rosato, M., et al., *Community participation: Lessons for maternal, newborn, and child health.* The Lancet, 2008. **372**(9642): p. 962–971.

96 Labonte, R., *Heart health inequalities in Canada: Modules, theory and planning.* Health Promotion International, 1992. **7**(2): p. 119–128.

97 Labonté, R., K. Mohindra, and T. Schrecker, *The growing impact of globalization for health and public health practice.* Annual Review of Public Health, 2011. **32**: p. 263–283.

98 Labonté, R., et al., *Globalization and health: Pathways, evidence and policy.* 2009: Routledge, London.

99 Blas, E. and A.S. Kurup, *Equity, social determinants and public health programmes.* 2010: World Health Organization, Geneva.

100 Blas, E., et al., *Social determinants approaches to public health: From concept to practice.* 2011: World Health Organization, Geneva.

101 Bandyopadhyay, M., *Tackling complexities in understanding the social determinants of health: The contribution of ethnographic research.* BMC Public Health, 2011. **11**(Suppl 5): p. S6.

102 Gjerdingen, D.K., D.G. Froberg, and P. Fontaine, *The effects of social support on women's health during pregnancy, labor and delivery, and the postpartum period.* Family Medicine, 1991. **23**(5): p. 370–375.

103 Tarkka, M.T. and M. Paunonen, *Social support and its impact on mothers' experiences of childbirth.* Journal of Advanced Nursing, 1996. **23**(1): p. 70–75.

104 Callister, L.C., *Cultural Meanings of Childbirth.* Journal of Obstetric, Gynaecologic and Neonatal Nursing, 1995. **24**(4): p. 327–331.

105 Alp, K.Ö. and M. Özdemir, *The tradition of presenting gold gifts after giving birth in Anatolia.* Folk Life, 2010. **48**(1): p. 35–47.

106 Veale, D., K. Furman, and D. Oliver, *South African traditional herbal medicines used during pregnancy and childbirth.* Journal of Ethnopharmacology, 1992. **36**(3): p. 185–191.

107 Douglas, M., *Purity and danger: An analysis of conception of body and pollution.* 1991: Routledge, London.

108 Douglas, M., *Risk and Blame: An analysis of concepts of pollution and taboo.* 1992: Routledge, London.

109 Douglas, M., *Purity and danger: An analysis of concepts of pollution and taboo.* 2003: Routledge, London.

110 Conrad, P. and K.K. Barker, *The Social Construction of Illness: Key Insights and Policy Implications.* Journal of Health and Social Behavior, 2010. **51**(1): p. S67–S79.

111 Walsh, D.J., *Childbirth embodiment: Problematic aspects of current understandings.* Sociology of Health and Illness, 2010. **32**(3): p. 486–501.

112 Banks, M., et al., *Risk and trust in the cultural industries.* Geoforum, 2000. **31**(4): p. 453–464.

113 Downe, S., *Campaign for normal birth. Trust and expertise.* RCM midwives: The Official Journal of the Royal College of Midwives, 2007. **10**(2): p. 66.

114 Downe, S., K. Finlayson, and A. Fleming, *Creating a collaborative culture in maternity care.* Journal of Midwifery and Women's Health, 2010. **55**(3): p. 250–254.

115 Oakley, A., *Women confined: Towards a sociology of childbirth.* 1980: Schocken, New York.

116 Boucher, D., et al., *Staying home to give birth: Why women in the United States choose home birth.* Journal of Midwifery and Women's Health, 2009. **54**(2): p. 119–126.

117 Leedam, E., *Traditional birth attendants.* International Journal of Gynaecology and Obstetrics, 1985. **23**(4): p. 249–274.

118 Hodnett, E., et al., *Continuous support for women during childbirth.* Birth, 2005. **32**(1): p. 72–72.

119 Hodnett, E.D., et al., *Continuous support for women during childbirth.* Cochrane Database of Systematic Reviews, 2013(7).

120 Crowther, S. and J. Hall, *Spirituality and spiritual care in and around childbirth.* Women and birth, 2015. **28**(2): p. 173–178.

121 Downe, S. and C. McCourt, *From being to becoming: Reconstructing childbirth.* Normal Childbirth E-Book: Evidence and Debate, 2008: Churchill Livingstone, London.

122 Kitzinger, S., *Authoritative touch in childbirth: A cross-cultural approach.* 1997: University of California Press, Oakland.

123 Kitzinger, S., *Some cultural perspectives of birth.* British Journal of Midwifery, 2000. **8**(12): p. 746–750.

124 Oakley, A., *Childbirth practice should take women's wishes into account.* BMJ: British Medical Journal, 1996. **313**(7071): p. 1557.

125 Douglas, M. and A. Wildavsky, *Risk and culture: An essay on the selection of technological and environmental dangers.* 1983: University of California Press, Oakland.

126 Giddens, A., *Risk, trust, reflexivity.* Reflexive Modernization. 1994: Polity Press, Cambridge. p. 184–197.

127 Giddens, A., *Risk and responsibility.* 1999: Blackwell Publishers, Oxford.

128 Armstrong, R., et al., *The role and theoretical evolution of knowledge translation and exchange in public health.* Journal of Public Health, 2006. **28**(4): p. 384–389.

129 Williams, G. and J. Popay, *Lay knowledge and the privilege of experience*. Challenging Medicine. 1994: Routledge, London. p. 118–139.

130 Adam, B., et al., *The risk society and beyond: Critical issues for social theory*. 2000: Sage Publications, Thousand Oaks.

131 Beck, U., *Risk society: Towards a new modernity*. 1992: Sage Publications, Thousand Oaks.

132 Mulinari, D. and K. Sandell, *A feminist re-reading of theories of late modernity: Beck, Giddens and the location of gender*. Critical Sociology, 2009. **35**(4): p. 493–507.

133 Horton-Salway, M. and A. Locke, *'But you might be damaging your baby': Constructing choice and risk in labour and childbirth*. Feminism and Psychology, 2010. **20**(4): p. 435–453.

134 Scammell, J. and D. Tait, *Using humanising values to support care*. Nursing Times, 2014. **110**(15): p. 16–18.

135 Luhmann, N., *Trust and power*. 2018: Wiley, Hoboken.

136 Giddens, A., *Modernity and self-identity: Self and society in the late modern age*. 1991: Stanford University Press, Redwood City.

137 Crotty, M., *The foundations of social research: Meaning and perspective in the research process*. 1998: Sage Publications, Thousand Oaks.

138 Goffman, E., *Frame analysis: An essay on the organization of experience*. 1974: Harvard University Press, Cambridge.

139 Blumer, H., *Symbolic interactionism: Perspective and method*. 1986: University of California Press, Oakland.

140 Sarantakos, S., *Social research*. 2012: Macmillan International Higher Education, London.

141 Newton, N. and M. Mead, Pregnancy, childbirth, and outcome: A review of patterns of culture and future research needs, in *Childbearing-its social and psychological aspects*. 1967: Williams and Wilkins, Baltimore.

142 LeCompte, M.D. and J.J. Schensul, *Analysis and interpretation of ethnographic data: A mixed methods approach*. Vol. 5. 2012: Rowman & Littlefield, Lanham.

143 Lock, A. and T. Strong, *Social constructionism: Sources and stirrings in theory and practice*. 2010: Cambridge University Press, Cambridge.

144 Lee-Rife, S.M., *Women's empowerment and reproductive experiences over the life course*. Social Science and Medicine, 2010. **71**(3): p. 634–642.

145 Edwards, R. *Connecting method and epistemology: A white women interviewing black women*. in *Women's Studies International Forum*. 1990: Elsevier, Amsterdam.

146 Agger, B., *Critical social theories*. 2006: ERIC, New York.

147 Tritten, J., *Giving voice to wisdom*. Midwifery Today and Childbirth Education, 1992. **2**(23): p. 3.

148 World Health Organisation, *Newborns: Reducing mortality fact sheet*. 2016: The World Health Organisation, Geneva.

149 Bennett, L., D.R. Dahal, and P. Govindasamy, *Caste, ethnic, and regional identity in Nepal: Further analysis of the 2006 Nepal Demographic and Health Survey*. 2008: Ministry of Health and Population, Government of Nepal, Kathmandu.

150 Bennett, L., *Gender, caste and ethnic exclusion in Nepal: Following the policy process from analysis to action*. 2005: The World Bank, Boston.

151 Dawson, P., et al., *From research to national expansion: 20 years' experience of community-based management of childhood pneumonia in Nepal*. Bulletin of the World Health Organization, 2008. **86**: p. 339–343.

152 Glenton, C., et al., *The female community health volunteer programme in Nepal: Decision makers' perceptions of volunteerism, payment and other incentives.* Social Science and Medicine, 2010. **70**(12): p. 1920–1927.

153 Lewin, S., et al., *Supporting the delivery of cost-effective interventions in primary health-care systems in low-income and middle-income countries: An overview of systematic reviews.* The Lancet, 2008. **372**(9642): p. 928–939.

154 Bennett, L., D. Dahal, and P. Govindasamy, *Caste, ethnic and regional identity in Nepal: Further analysis of the 2006 Nepal demographic and health survey. 2008.* 2018: Macro International Inc, Calverton.

155 Gagnon, A., et al., *Obstetrical complications associated with abnormal maternal serum markers analytes.* Journal of Obstetrics and Gynaecology Canada, 2008. **30**(10): p. 918–932.

156 Murshed, S.M. and S. Gates, *Spatial – horizontal inequality and the Maoist insurgency in Nepal.* Review of Development Economics, 2005. **9**(1): p. 121–134.

157 Regmi, K. *Childbirth practices in Nepal: A review of models for reducing adverse outcomes.* International Journal of Gynaecology and Obstetrics, 2009. **107**(2): p. 321.

158 Regmi, K., R. Smart, and J. Kottler, *Understanding gender and power dynamics within the family: A qualitative study of Nepali women's experience.* Australian and New Zealand Journal of Family Therapy, 2010. **31**(2): p. 191–201.

159 Adhikari, R., *Demographic, socio-economic, and cultural factors affecting fertility differentials in Nepal.* BMC Pregnancy and Childbirth, 2010. **10**(1): p. 19.

160 Lee, A.C., et al., *Community-based stillbirth rates and risk factors in rural Sarlahi, Nepal.* International Journal of Gynaecology and Obstetrics, 2011. **113**(3): p. 199–204.

161 Shahabuddin, A., et al., *Determinants of institutional delivery among young married women in Nepal: Evidence from the Nepal demographic and health survey, 2011.* BMJ Open, 2017. **7**(4): p. e012446.

162 Shrestha, B.P., et al., *Community interventions to reduce child mortality in Dhanusha, Nepal: Study protocol for a cluster randomized controlled trial.* Trials, 2011. **12**(1): p. 1–14.

163 Shrestha, M. and S. Shrestha, *Women's Role in Nepal in General and Population Control in particular-An Assessment.* Tribhuvan University Journal, 1991. **14**: p. 27–41.

164 Pokharel, S., *Gender discriminatory practices in Tamang and Brahmin communities.* Tribhuvan University Journal, 2009. **26**(1): p. 85–98.

165 Bhandari, A., M. Gordon, and G. Shakya, *Reducing maternal mortality in Nepal.* BJOG: An International Journal of Obstetrics and Gynaecology, 2011. **118**(s2): p. 26–30.

166 Ahmed, M., et al., *Utilization of rural maternity delivery services in Nawalparasi and Kapilvastu District: A Qualitative Study.* Journal of College of Medical Sciences Nepal, 2010. **6**(3): p. 29–36.

167 Brunson, J., *Son preference in the context of fertility decline: limits to new constructions of gender and kinship in Nepal.* Studies in Family Planning, 2010. **41**(2): p. 89–98.

168 Maitra, P., *Effect of socioeconomic characteristics on age at marriage and total fertility in Nepal.* Journal of Health, Population and Nutrition, 2004: p. 84–96.

169 Pandey, J.P., *Maternal and child health in Nepal: The effects of caste, ethnicity, and regional identity: Further analysis of the 2011 Nepal demographic and health survey.* 2013: Ministry of Health and Population, Kathmandu.

170 Basnyat, I., *Beyond biomedicine: Health through social and cultural understanding.* Nursing Inquiry, 2011. **18**(2): p. 123–134.

171 Simkhada, B., M.A. Porter, and E.R. Van Teijlingen, *The role of mothers-in-law in antenatal care decision-making in Nepal: A qualitative study*. BMC Pregnancy and Childbirth, 2010. **10**(1): p. 34.

172 Subedi, M., *Caste system: Theories and practices in Nepal*. Himalayan Journal of Sociology and Anthropology, 2010. **4**(3): p. 134–159.

173 Christie, M.E. and K. Giri, *Challenges and experiences of women in the forestry sector in Nepal*. International Journal of Sociology and Anthropology, 2011. **3**(5): p. 139–146.

174 Jackson, M.A., *Empowering women of Nepal: An experience of empowerment in the land of the Himalaya*. 2010: Prescott College, Arizona.

175 Kaufman, M.R. and M. Crawford, *Research and activism review: Sex trafficking in Nepal: A review of intervention and prevention programs*. Violence Against Women, 2011. **17**(5): p. 651–665.

176 Adhikari, R. and Y. Sawangdee, *Influence of women's autonomy on infant mortality in Nepal*. Reproductive Health, 2011. **8**(1): p. 7.

177 Brunson, J., *Confronting maternal mortality, controlling birth in Nepal: The gendered politics of receiving biomedical care at birth*. Social Science and Medicine, 2010. **71**(10): p. 1719–1727.

178 Bryers, H.M. and E. Van Teijlingen, *Risk, theory, social and medical models: A critical analysis of the concept of risk in maternity care*. Midwifery, 2010. **26**(5): p. 488–496.

179 Poudel, P., *Pregnancy outcomes in Nepal: An investigation of the relationships between socioeconomic factors, maternal factors and foetal and maternal outcomes in a Pokhara sample: A thesis presented in partial fulfilment of the requirements for the degree of Master of Arts in Nursing at Massey University*. 1999: Massey University, Palmerston North.

2   Socio-cultural perspective of childbirth

Introduction

Dolma lives about a day and half walk from the district hospital. She was married at the age of 14. Dolma and her family follow Buddhism, but their practice is mixed with Hindu tradition. She started her childbirth journey at the age of 16. She is now 35 years old and this is her 10th pregnancy. So far, she has gone through one miscarriage, one stillbirth, two newborn deaths and one of her children died at the age of three. Dolma gave birth to all her children in the corner of her house. Her four children living with her are currently aged between three to nine years and she is expecting another one in a week or two. She has no plan to leave home. For Dolma, the corner of the house is the safest place to experience birth.

Childbirth has significant social and cultural meaning in Nepal [1, 2]. Culture and tradition vary from one place to another, but childbirth is often considered as a universal experience [3]. Even though childbirth follows the same physiological process, different communities interpret that experience differently [4]. Their meaning of childbirth is based on the interaction of social and cultural factors to construct the experience. The way women living in urban areas describes childbirth is different to the way women living in rural areas does in Nepal [1, 5, 6]. This difference is further explained by inequalities in service utilisation during childbirth resulting in more deaths in rural and remote communities.

Women living in both Western and non-Western cultures situate their childbirth experiences within the context of their lives [7–9]. Socio-cultural systems and embedded relationships play an important role in women's childbirth experiences [10, 11]. This concept of relationship is vital to examine in making sense of childbirth experiences. According to Oakley [12], culture provides a set of norms that influence attitudes, values, views and interpretations of childbirth in different societies. It is important to acknowledge that women living in culturally rich settings see childbirth as a socially constructed event and their meaning of childbirth evolves around their values, tradition and cultural practice. Callister et al. [13] outline the influences of socio-cultural values, beliefs and practices on motherhood experience which commence with childbirth. Steinberg [14] exemplifies this view by considering childbirth as a part of women's daily household chores. In rural and remote Nepal, childbirth is a normal and ongoing task for women [2, 6, 15].

Certain cultural practices help to create safety in women's childbirth experiences [16–19]. For example, traditions of helping women by providing warmth and massage by experienced female relatives or traditional birth attendants (TBAs) during the birth contribute to promoting safety during childbirth [20–24]. Socio-cultural view disagrees with the concept of childbirth as an individual physiological experience requiring only medical interventions and consistently argues to consider the social context of women when it comes to childbirth [2].

Lupton [25] criticises medicine for not considering childbirth as a part of the social and cultural life of women. Further criticism is made how the Western medical view considers socio-cultural environments as risks for adverse health outcomes during childbirth forcing women to give birth in institutional settings [26–28]. Using risk-based messaging and asking women to come to healthcare facilities to give birth has been the biggest policy attempt in South Asian countries including Nepal. Women who do not use medical services during childbirth are often blamed by healthcare providers for causing maternal and newborn deaths [1, 2, 5, 29]. In spite of this, many Nepalese women prefer giving birth within their community [2, 30].

The socio-cultural situation in Nepal is often considered as a barrier to accessing medical services to prevent childbirth-related deaths. Bennett et al. [31] argue that the childbirth tradition in Nepal prevails negatively on maternal, newborn and child health. Thapa et al. [32] further comment that the culture often prevents women from accessing essential healthcare services resulting in higher maternal and newborn mortality. Dahal [33] portrays the social practice of giving birth in the cowshed as a risk producing task. Schubert et al. [34] claim childbirth pollution as the cause of adverse birth outcomes. Nevertheless, the value that rural Nepalese women give to culture and tradition to gain childbirth safety during childbirth outweigh the use of medical services. Available evidence confirms that the meaning of childbirth for remote mountain women is culturally constructed and socially transformed over the years.

Authority of childbirth knowledge

There are two forms of knowledge: one is expert or scientific knowledge and the other is lay or traditional knowledge [35–37]. Taking traditional knowledge into account allows better understanding of childbirth experiences of women in cross-cultural settings. Drawing on Popay and Williams [38], considering the place of lay knowledge provides a basis of understanding tradition, social practice and its impact on childbirth experiences of women in a number of ways. Firstly, awareness of lay knowledge can provide a more nuanced understanding of the factors contributing to childbirth. Secondly, the incorporation of lay knowledge around the childbirth risks can contribute to better understanding of the causes of associated morbidity and mortality. Lastly, when subjective experiences of childbirth are not confirmed by more objective measures, the medical construction of risks and safety takes over the personal experiences.

Nevertheless, incorporating lived experiences of women with recognition of the impacts of structural factors is critical to the creation and authority of childbirth knowledge. The concept of lay knowledge is significant for understanding people's experiences because in many cultures traditional knowledge is valued more than the medical knowledge [36]. Sociologists provided consistent arguments for giving importance to lay knowledge to control the birthing process and to experience childbirth [39–41]. Feminist writers argue that the use of traditional or Indigenous knowledge is paramount in ensuring childbirth safety [7, 42–44]. In their view, safety entails women's ownership and control of the childbirth process, without medical and technological interference.

In South Asia, knowledge creation is influenced by culture, tradition, religion and people's inherited faith system [45]. Once knowledge is formed, it is passed on to other generations by elders. The same process occurs while creating and sharing childbirth knowledge. In Hindu and Buddhist mythologies, physical suffering that women experience during childbirth is a normal part of life. God has a significant place in making meaning of women's childbirth experiences in South Asia. Mostly, their knowledge of childbirth is based on how the family and society value God.

The real meaning of childbirth can be understood by considering the socio-cultural context in which it occurs. In rural Nepal, traditional knowledge about childbirth influences the decision on where and how to give birth and the care of mother and newborn [46–50]. Women trust traditions more and prefer their mother-in-law or other village women to help without the fears of being victim of medicalised care which consider childbirth as a risky event [2, 51]. The socio-cultural view of childbirth allows women to exercise both the authority and power of their traditional knowledge to take ownership of their experience. Women's trust in traditional knowledge is an important aspect of childbirth safety in cross-cultural communities.

The Western medical view gives authority to medical knowledge to control childbirth. The medical model views women as birth machines and obstetricians, physicians and nurses as the mechanics to operate a women's body as they wish [52–54]. This is not the way women want or like to be treated while experiencing a significant event in their life. In an institutional setting, women have limited opportunity to resist medical authority while giving birth and this means their interests and preferences are not acknowledged [55–57]. Sadly, many women are institutionalised to give birth as it is considered mandatory to minimise the risk [58–62]. This situation is apparent because most health services are biomedically informed that often devalue the traditional birth practice and disempower women during childbirth.

The authority of medical knowledge does not only separate women from their socio-cultural setting, but it also ignores women as subjects of their birthing experiences [60, 63–65]. Furthermore, the blame is rampant to women and their helpers get blamed for being irrational and incapable of managing medical risks during childbirth [66, 67]. Because of the fear of death created by the medical model, women tend to remain silent and place their confidence in the doctor [68]. The authority of medical knowledge has controlled the childbirth experiences of women. Consequently, this authority of knowledge and control of the birthing process is creating threats to the safety of women living in the culturally rich setting of South Asia. This has led to women opting not to seek help from healthcare workers or going to hospital to give birth.

Critical feminism values everyday life situations while considering the meaning of childbirth and considers women as the experts in their experiences. It describes medical domination in childbirth as oppression to gain safety during childbirth [69]. When knowledge develops through experiences, it is more authentic [70]. The knowledge women create from their everyday life experiences is valued in feminist research. Similarly, social constructionism assumes that knowledge is constructed through social interactions, influences and relationships [71]. These perspectives provide a framework to understand and make meaning of women's lived experiences.

Nepalese women living in rural areas give authority to traditional knowledge and accept non-professional support to give birth within their community [6, 20]. Even women living in urban areas have expressed dissatisfaction with the control of medical professionals while giving birth in hospital [1, 5]. The reliance on traditional healing systems in rural areas of Nepal demonstrates trust and confidence in the lay knowledge [24, 59, 72]. In the context of remote mountains, authority is given to the traditional knowledge where women prefer staying in the village to experience birth.

Ownership of childbirth experiences

Social constructionism and critical feminism theories give ownership of experiences to the people [73]. These theories talk about two different forms of ownership: one is individual and the other is collective. Agreeing with other sociologists [7, 39, 52–54, 74–77], childbirth is a shared social experience which gives collective ownership to women living in cross-cultural communities. Having a choice to decide the birthing place gives ownership of the childbirth experience to women [17, 78–82]. This ownership of experiences is developed through the ability to control the birthing process and women's feeling of safety during the birth. Women giving birth in institutional settings have little or no control over to the experiences of giving birth [6]. The socio-cultural perspective of childbirth values the significance of giving ownership of childbirth experiences to women, so it becomes an empowering journey.

Lived and subjective experiences of individuals are socially constructed [83]. For many Nepalese women, childbirth is a social event where knowledge, support, resources and outcomes are shared within the community [2, 5]. When help is needed, older women (either the mother-in-law or other neighbouring women from the village) are called to assist the birth [2, 24]. In this instance, both women and the helpers work together to control and manage the birthing process and take ownership of the experiences.

When childbirth occurs in an institutional setting, the power to control the process goes to the medical professionals and these women become powerless [17, 84–86]. Childbirth then becomes a physiological condition requiring technical interventions keeping women in a controlled environment with no opportunity to be part of the birthing process [87, 88]. As a result, rural women in many countries tend to avoid hospitals and remain home to give birth [89–91]. As childbirth is a part of women's lives, it should not be taken away from them [92]. However, in rural Nepal, it is family members rather than the woman who makes decisions about where and how to give birth [1, 5, 93]. In that sense, childbirth is a collective experience of women, family, and community members [94–96]. While women help other women, their experiences are built through the influences of relationships and interactions which contribute to the collective ownership of the birth.

Risky or safe: choices in childbirth

Mansfield [97] demonstrates the crucial influence of relationships in the birth experience of women. Continuous support of family members and other known persons have been found to be beneficial to women while giving birth [88, 98]. Relationships with the support person and caregivers play a critical role at childbirth. Thus, relationships are one of the major components of childbirth safety. Callister [13, 99] places emphasis on cultural and spiritual dimensions of safety in a cross-cultural setting. For Douglas [76, 100], safety focuses on maintaining childbirth knowledge, beliefs, traditions and practices of a socio-cultural setting. This view of safety, also known as a culturalist view, considers the influences of social circumstances and relationships in childbirth experiences of women.

In the socio-cultural perspective, safety is a perception that helps to examine the influences of social relationships on childbirth. Douglas [100] argues that how safety is perceived depends on which social and cultural group the person belongs to. The perceived sense of safety varies according to a person's social values and their cultural belief system [78, 80, 101–105]. Safety emphasises two major themes: first, concerning the different types of knowledge which inform the perception of safety, and second, the moral dimension of safety [106, 107]. Different people have different forms of relationships which can influence their perception of safety. In practice, focusing on cultural and spiritual safety promotes satisfaction and ownership of childbirth experiences [108–113]. How safety is viewed, constructed and practiced during childbirth could be different according to the cultural setting.

The social, embodied and discursive constraints on women's agency in the context of a medically dominated birthing practice compromise the rhetoric of "choice" and limit the women's ability to maintain independent agency by the set of clinical procedures. Choice in childbirth is associated with the individual autonomy and responsibility to make informed decisions. The notion of choice is influenced by the agency and structure. Agency here refers to an individual's capacity to act independently and to make free choices; where structure refers to those factors that restrict opportunities to make those choices [114]. Walsh [11] pointed to a tension between personal agency and social structure when it comes to childbirth because the structural factors such as social class, gender, religion, ethnicity, culture, tradition, system and process play critical roles while making decisions about where and how to give birth.

The choice in the structuralist view attempts to overcome the division between structure and personal agency by emphasising influence of the nature of circumstances [115]. Giddens highlights the productive role that person plays in maintaining and recreating social codes and norms. For Giddens, this process of recreation helps to transform the structure so individuals can make free choices. In this view, people deploy practical consciousness during their lives to sustain or transform the structural components of their society. This concept provides safe grounding to analyse what components of a social system are in the interest of participants to continue and what need transformation and how changes can be made when required. This requires both individual and social agencies working together to create structures that will determine what choices women can make about childbirth.

There have been constant sociological critiques to the medical concept risk in childbirth. The term risk consistently refers to birth-related problems and outcomes. The perception of risk is a major component of the childbirth experience which influences the way women view childbirth and their choices of birthplace and support person [116]. Even today, the birthing process in biomedicine is grounded with metaphors of risk in which professional control and medical interventions become a routine strategy. The common practice of taking women away from their community or not allowing them to use their traditional practices hinders safety [42, 117].

The medical risk epistemology divides pregnant women into "high-risk" and "low-risk" categories [1]. The risk categorisation assumes that the obstetric model is better for high-risk women and the midwifery model of care can be an option for low-risk women [118, 119]. The medical risk approach has childbirth as an individual experience and is limited to understand the impact of socio-cultural factors critical to women.

The social view of risk focuses on cultural, emotional and spiritual safety during childbirth. Beck [120, 121] ties social risk implicitly to reflexive modernisation and argues that the wider environmental and social risks are a product of techno-scientific interventions which creates a threat to safety. The "Risks Society" [120] claims that our own production and technologies produce risks. In that sense, society and many technologies including medicine are risk producers. Giddens [122] adds to the creation of risks because of the danger and uncertainties that the world is facing currently. This supports the argument that medical knowledge, associated technologies and clinical interventions produce other risks to women during childbirth.

Beck [120] and Giddens [122] argue that the medical notion of risks often demands experts' identification and calculation making others follow special measures to understand the nature of risks and how to manage them. Lupton [106] supports the argument and goes further confirming that the expert's judgement of risk can create threats and uncertainties in childbirth. Unlike the medical risk approach, the lay view of risk is supported by the cultural and symbolic approach which considers risk as a part of shared understanding and practices [100, 123–125]. Douglas's view on risk stems from the cultural meaning of childbirth associated with the notion of purity, pollution and otherness important to certain cultural groups. Lupton [66, 106, 107] supports Douglas's view and emphasises how the community develops cultural strategy to understand the external threats coming to them and takes appropriate actions to maintain social cohesion and stability. Thus, the perceptions of risk are based on the social and cultural factors which are imminent to understand the meaning of childbirth and how women develop their sense of safety.

Power and empowerment in childbirth

Discussion about childbirth in the cross-cultural setting of South Asia requires one to unpack the context of power. Many relationships that influence the childbirth experience of women revolves around the power of dynamics. Unequal distribution of power in relation to gender, ethnicity, income status, social class, locations and many other factors has been considered as a major obstacle to address the health gap globally [126, 127]. The exercise of power is not only an action of domination or control but also turns out to consist of the manipulation of thoughts, attitudes and social relationships [128]. This construct of power has major influence in ownership and control of childbirth experiences.

The most common form of power is legitimate power which is defined as the authority that individuals hold in family and society [129]. Another form of power is referent power which is defined as individuals having the ability to be a frame of reference and serve in the role of a significant other [130]. Men's legitimacy being highly evident in South Asian societies where women hold a higher level of referent power. Because of the strong influence of Hinduism in South Asia, patriarchy and patriarchal norms are deeply rooted in society which has had a profound effect on women and their childbirth experiences. Patriarchy has an intergenerational effect on women in South Asia: daughters are expected to be under the control of the father, as a wife of her husband and as a widow of her son. Some Hindu codes place women as "Goddess" which allows them to practice reference power on special occasions, but the influence of patriarchy is higher when it comes to power. These forms of power create more complexities for women to understand their own status and power.

The other form of power is expert power which is a social power brought into a relationship, through education, knowledge, skills and experience [131]. This type of power has high relevance to childbirth in terms of making decisions about the place, support person and process. The form and authority of childbirth knowledge are determined by the expert power in the medical model where health professionals control the birthing process. In cross-cultural social settings, the expertise lies with the person that women have relationships and trust to be part of their childbirth experiences. Using stories of women, I will provide a thorough analysis of how this power relationship works in the context of childbirth experiences of women living in the Himalayas.

Michael Foucault argues that power originates from everywhere and is involved in all human interactions [132, 133]. Foucault describes power and knowledge as interconnected concepts and argues that the shift from traditionalism to modernity in childbirth is a result of coercive power, which replaces the ideology of social relationships with technological interventions. In Foucault's view, childbirth in the medical model has been commoditised with the rise of monitoring technology, doctors and midwives are reduced to mechanics in the production process and women are treated as a passive object in the process. The medical process denies the role of relationships, cross-cultural values and social control of birth. Foucault's critical analysis of power further reinforced by Martin [134] as dominant medical metaphor in childbirth in relation to how the roles and relationships between providers and women tend to fit with the model which sees the doctor as manager, midwife as worker, mother as machine and baby as product. The analysis of power enables understanding of how childbirth knowledge is enacted and maintained or resisted and changed over the time.

Connell [129] identifies the influence of power dynamics on women's autonomy at both family and societal levels. Iris Marion Young develops related insights into the presence of coercive power even where overt force is absent [135]. She notes that oppression can designate, not only brutal tyranny over entire populations by a few rulers but also the disadvantage and injustice some people suffer because of the everyday practices of a well-intentioned liberal society. Young terms this "structural oppression," whose forms are systematically reproduced in major economic, political and cultural institutions [136]. Power can be also understood as a relation in which people are empowered through critical reflection leading to shared actions. Feminism sees collective action as power leading to a transformation of existing structures by creating alternative modes [114]. It has been confirmed that reducing social inequalities requires changes in the distribution of power and power relationships [137]. Understanding the context of power gives opportunity to examine the influences of various relationships that women have during childbirth.

Another concept consistently discussed in the context of health is empowerment which aims to enable people to create positive change [138]. Theoretically, there are multi-level constructs about empowerment representing both processes and outcomes for individual and community levels [139]. At the individual level, psychological empowerment illustrates the concept that includes people's perceived control in their lives, their critical awareness of their social environment and their participation in the change process [140]. Community-level processes include people's ability to work cross culturally as well as outcomes of transformed conditions [138]. From the PHC perspective, empowerment includes the process of enabling people, both individuals and groups, to gain control over their own affairs, by increasing their capacity to make choices and transform those choices into desired actions and outcomes [141].

Commonly defined concepts of empowerment involve a process by which people experience more control over the decisions that influence their health and lives [142]. This concept focuses on collective ownership and collective actions to enhance positive experiences and outcomes. Furthermore, Laverack [143] sees empowerment as a shift towards greater equality in the social relations of power. The empowerment emphasises community taking control of resources and being involved in the decision-making process to take necessary action. Empowerment mostly focuses on gaining power and ability in a way that increases self-efficacy and decision-making [144]. In childbirth, empowerment is associated with both psychological and social domains and aims to have a sense of control of the whole experience as well as a sense of involvement in the birth process.

In South Asia, the concept of female power (Shakti) is rooted with the ability to endure pain during childbirth. The pain during birth is considered normal and giving birth without any professional and medical interventions enhanced the sense of power. An empowering birthing experience for women characterised with the sense of being strengthened, enabled and authorised [144]. Women who can give birth in their chosen place with the support of a trusted person are most likely to feel empowered by their experiences. However, there are ongoing power interplays among women, service providers, caregivers and other people which tend to take away the sense of control from women [57, 145, 146]. In Nepal, there is a significant power dynamic apparent at the family and societal levels [2].

So, these different forms of power and different patterns of relationships influence childbirth decisions for women. Sometimes these make women powerless through their own experiences. However, at times, when women can be part of the process to decide where and how to give birth, their experience becomes empowering. Empowering childbirth facilitated by a positive family, care provider and social relationships contributes to having satisfactory experiences and helps women to maintain a sense of social, cultural and emotional safety.

Dynamics of gender and relationships in childbirth

The social construct of gender has significant influences on childbirth [2, 54, 74, 147, 148]. Gender is a socially constructed concept which sets characteristics, norms and roles for women and men. The influence of gendered relationships is often critical in the childbirth experiences of women [149–151]. In South Asian society, the nature of relationships is impacted by gendered social norms and the power distributions. The construct of gender creates standards for men and women to follow that somehow becomes critical in relationships to make choices and decisions. In Nepal, childbirth experiences of women depend highly on the nature of gendered family and societal relationships [1, 2, 152].

Feminist researchers examine how gendered relationships come into play in family and society to understand women's issues related to childbirth and motherhood [73, 153–156]. Morley and Macfarlane [95] consider gendered power relationships as a part of larger societal discourse that shape systems and practices and demand negotiation to create supportive influences. It is evident that childbirth is influenced by common social practices, cultural values and relationships in which gender and power come side by side [96].

Gendered divisions within society affect health through unequal distribution of power and responsibility whereby women's lower social status and lack of control over resources expose them to risk [157]. Gendered social norms in South Asia confines women to domestic responsibilities, limiting their opportunity to access educational and economic resources [158]. Gender-based discrimination, where girls and women get limited access to resources, opportunities and services, is rampant in many societies [159]. The gendered division of responsibilities and gender-based discrimination have direct impact on childbirth experiences of women. In addition, girls are expected to get married young to mature men in a traditional way and forced to get pregnant soon after the marriage [160]. This puts women at further risk of having poor pregnancy and birth outcomes.

In South Asia, gender discrimination is highly prevalent due to the patrilineal structure of society [161]. The male child has the right to property ownership in most South Asian countries. In Hindu society, many significant rituals are only allowed to perform by male members of the family. Giving birth to a male child is a tremendous pressure for women in these societies, which encourages them to go through multiple pregnancies. When the birth of male child happens in the family, it ends up being a grand celebration [2]. The birth of girl child is often neglected and the inability to give birth to a male child can lead to violence and emotional torture against women. Biologically, a greater survival rate is noted among girls, but this ratio in South Asian countries is different where boys have higher survival rates than girls in the age below six years [161]. Sadly, socially active patriarchy and gender-based discriminations rooted in society have disempowered women historically and the impacts of this is evident in their childbirth experiences.

The influence of family and societal relationships in childbirth experiences is discussed widely [40, 71, 103, 162, 163]. The role of family members, especially the mother-in-law, is critical to women during childbirth [1, 2]. The relationship is complex due to the power dynamics as the daughter-in-law has a submissive status whereas the mother-in-law holds a powerful status. In this scenario, women who give birth show both resistance and resentment in response to the unfair treatment they receive from their mothers-in-law [15]. The tensions and complexities of various relationships in childbirth are worth exploring to understand the meaning and the nature of childbirth experiences of women living in diverse social settings.

Structural influences in childbirth

Structural factors such as ethnicity, income, education and place of residence are associated with maternal and newborn deaths [9, 164–169]. The socio-cultural perspective of childbirth recognises the influence of these structural determinants in childbirth experiences of women [11, 71]. Several studies demonstrate the association of structural factors with birth outcomes demonstrating that Indigenous women, women with low-income status, women with low education status and remote-rural women are more likely to experience stillbirths and neonatal losses [170–174]. Socio-economic disparities in maternal and newborn health outcomes have been an ongoing challenge, and no effective policies have been introduced yet to address the issue. As a result, inequalities are widening, making rural and remote populations most vulnerable with limited access to resources, opportunities and services.

Unequal access to safe childbirth services is considered as one of the main reasons for socio-economic disparities in maternal and newborn health outcomes [175–178]. In Nepal, it has been recognised for decades that women living in the mountain districts have geographic difficulties in accessing quality maternal health services which has contributed to higher numbers of maternal and neonatal deaths [178, 179]. The distance to a hospital has been a predictor of poor utilisation of prenatal and childbirth services in rural areas of Nepal [180, 181]. So far, there have been limited attempts to address the wider determinants to ensure that every woman has easy access to information, resources and services to experience safe childbirth.

Women's educational attainment, social status, household economy and decision-making power have association with their healthcare seeking behaviour and childbirth-related survival in developing countries [182–187]. The socio-economic position of the individual including income, education, social class (gender and ethnicity) and occupation are critical factors creating inequities in health outcomes [137]. Arguments have been made to focus on increasing access to transport, food supply and other basic resources to promote health outcomes [188]. In Nepal, geographic inequity in distribution and availability of maternal and newborn health services limits opportunities for women living in remote and rural communities resulting in higher mortalities [189–191]. These structural determinants have direct influence in childbirth experiences of women who lack basic resources, services and opportunities.

Structural factors become barriers to women living in remote areas making them unable to exercise the same rights to health care as everyone else [192, 193]. These determinants influence women's autonomy to make decisions about childbirth, as women living in low resource settings have limited choices to make [170, 194]. Issues of poverty and casteism in South Asia are still a huge challenge leading to inadequate food and hunger for women and their families from low socio-economic backgrounds. These issues have created the social stratification with hierarchical power structure where people in lower socio-economic status (SES) have limited options and access to resources. This translates to childbirth experiences of women resulting in socio-economic inequalities in birth outcomes. Identifying, acknowledging and examining the impacts of structural determinants to childbirth experiences of women living in remote mountain areas of Nepal will provide deeper insights to how the context of their living impacts birth outcomes.

Culture, tradition and spirituality in childbirth

The socio-cultural perspective of childbirth acknowledges culture and traditions as the key aspects of women's life and plays an influential role in childbirth experiences. In many cultures, including those of South Asia, childbirth is considered as an untouchable and impure event [15, 29, 32, 195]. Women are kept in isolation after the birth of their baby for up to 30 days. In some cultures, bleeding after childbirth is considered normal to clear the impurities from a woman's body [196]. In cultures where childbirth is a highly traditional event, women prefer giving birth within their community [2, 80, 123, 197]. South Asian women experience childbirth in a highly traditional fashion. In rural Nepal, women are being consigned to the Goth (animal shed) to give birth and to spend their polluted postnatal days [2, 32, 198]. The length of period and principles of seclusion vary between different groups and communities across different countries. Once the specific period is over, family often holds a purifying ritual to accept women back to normal life.

Every society has cultural practices, traditions, belief systems and rituals related to childbirth. These can set the norms for family to follow in terms of what women can do and what is restricted to do before or after childbirth. The place of culture and tradition remains strongly even for those who are educated and exposed with a modern environment. So, the use of TBAs to help women giving birth is a common practice in many rural villages in South Asia [199–201]. These attendants are traditional, non-formally trained, independent, locally trusted and a community-based support person for women during pregnancy, childbirth and the postnatal period [202]. Women's preference for using these TBAs is linked with easy access and trust in the traditional knowledge and the minimal cost [20, 181, 203]. The traditional birthing model has been used widely in many communities because this provides personalised emotional support and is sensitive to the economic and socio-cultural preferences of women [2, 204]. In rural and remote communities even when medically trained care providers are available, women have more trust in the experienced local women or TBAs to seek help while giving birth [24, 30, 205].

Childbirth is a spiritually and religiously significant life event for many women. The dominance of medicalised childbirth has been questioned consistently, as it remains emotionally and spiritually unsatisfying for many women and their families [206]. There are obvious intersections between religion, spirituality and childbirth. For some women, childbirth is a spiritually moving and sacred experience in which the restrictions of not being able to perform certain rituals threaten their emotional safety [80]. Ritual and symbolic aspects of healing are profoundly important in Indigenous childbirth practice. In an Australian study, Aboriginal women collectively express their desire to maintain cultural practice by giving birth in their country with the involvement of family and a trusted support worker [207]. Another study confirms that failing to incorporate Indigenous knowledge and practice of childbirth in the Western medical model has created a sense of cultural insecurity among Koori women in South-Eastern Australia [208]. A cultural birthing area has high significance in the Aboriginal community which involves a birthing tree or birthing cave. Aboriginal women describe birthing trees as ceremonial places that connect newborn to ancestors and the country [110]. Birthing women use the branch of a birthing tree to relieve the pain during birth [208]. Like a birthing tree, the birthing caves are believed to be a sacred place to connect the soul with the country and hold cultural significance of birthing practice. There are other rituals and beliefs that Aboriginal women prefer to continue and maintain the cultural safety of childbirth [110].

Religion and spirituality have significant influence to construct the meaning of childbirth and to shape birthing practices Nepal [209–211]. Communities link causes of childbirth-related problems or deaths with supernatural powers [210, 212]. Thus, Traditional Faith Healers are invited to perform rituals to overcome the threats to survival of mothers and babies [212–214]. The Hindu religion positions women as the subordinates to men [93, 215]. This limits the opportunities of making decisions about life matters including childbirth for women of Hindu society. Religion further discriminates between societies within the caste system where women from the lower caste category are more disadvantaged and have limited access to information, resources and services [31, 216].

Oppression to liberation: a critical dialogue in childbirth

Women in South Asia are conditioned to perform as a good wife, daughter-in-law and mother, as these roles require qualities such as the suppressing of self-desire and embracing of self-sacrifice, staying silent and following the expectations set to them. The notion of femininity and masculinity in the patriarchal structure sees socially constructed roles as normal, and thus women are expected to be controlled by men. However, the male control and power is associated with the continued oppression of women in society which manifests inequalities in many aspects of life. Women are not only experiencing social control due to the deep-rooted patriarchy but also being politically oppressed while not having voices or choices in the decision-making process. This results in multiple forms of oppression which requires action beyond the social structure to make childbirth an empowering experience for women.

Feminist philosophy is committed to overcoming oppression resulting from unequal social relations specifically those related to gender [217, 218]. In other words, the commitment to the emancipation of women is central in critical feminism. The central themes of critical feminism include inclusiveness, cooperation and collaboration, mutual respect and trust, multiple ways of knowing and collective action that challenges the marginalisation and the silencing of women [218]. Given that childbirth is predominantly related to women, critical feminism can be a meaningful and enlightening approach to enhance a positive experience for women. This approach offers the opportunity to analyse the diversity of childbirth experiences of women and associated issues of power and oppression [219]. Similarly, the central tenets of empowerment and transformation in critical feminism allow women to claim ownership of their pregnancy and childbirth experiences.

Critical feminism draws on the concept of oppression and allows one to understand the exclusion of women in the form of gender, social class, race, ethnicity and education (Weedon, 1997). Attempts to contextualise the marginality of women involve examining the social positioning of women within the given structure and agency which construct the power to influence everyday practice. I argue that the feminist analysis of gender should not only focus on the criticism of patriarchy or the power clash between men and women, but it should also take other social factors into the account to understand how the power is constructed, gained and operated within society. Critical feminist researchers use reflexivity by engaging participants in understanding and emancipation, allowing reflection about their lives, raising consciousness, making the oppressive nature of women's circumstances evident to others and acting for liberation [220]. In childbirth, this focuses on giving women power to control their experiences to decide where and how they want to give birth. Making childbirth a liberating experience for women requires a critical approach.

Freire's [221, 222] critical pedagogy, particularly his "Pedagogy of the Oppressed," rests upon the vision of social transformation through liberation and opposition to oppression, which is also the central focus of critical feminism. The critical pedagogy that Freire develops focuses on concepts of oppression, conscientisation and dialogue. Freire gives value to collective knowledge and action. Central to Freire's pedagogy is the practice of conscientisation that is coming to the consciousness of oppression and the commitment to end that oppression. To end the oppression, Freire offers an approach which instigates dialogue between the oppressors and the oppressed. In this dialogical approach, the assumption is that the oppressors are on the same side of the oppressed and that they engage together in a dialogue about the world. The dialogue between them uncovers the same reality, the same oppression and the same liberation, which he calls collective liberation. This collective liberation is what the critical feminist theorists are also aiming for to give women ownership of their experiences.

Iris Marion Young [136] explains about the different nature of relationships and power interplays within and outside the social structure. Young further argues that people deny the differences and do not trust or respect people they do not know. Therefore, people strive for mutual identification, shared understanding and reciprocity [135]. Young talks about five faces of oppression: violence, exploitation, marginalisation, powerlessness and cultural imperialism currently existed in society. From a political philosophical point of view, Young highlights the existing inequalities and envisions a society which denies oppression, values reciprocity of understanding, fosters social relations of equality and shares common values. Young argues that mediating with the people who are not parts of the community and who share their differences makes it possible to create a good society, which in her term is an "unoppressive city."

Heath [223] introduces the concept of collaborative dialogue and suggests three different dialogic themes in relation to collaboration. First, Heath argues that dialogue generates new ideas, thoughts, processes and outcomes. Second, Heath acknowledges the diversity of ideas and argues for community dialogue and creativity which can contribute to negotiating differences elicited by diversity. Third, Heath argues that dialogue allows for reciprocity and symmetry between participants in which power is shared and negotiated in decision-making situations. In line with Freire [221], Heath argues that dialogue enables participants to share their ideas and negotiate power in their relationships which raises consciousness and leads to transformative and more liberating relationships. Consistent with Young [136], Heath argues further that dialogue allows the conditions to be built that can counter the talk and action that silences community voices, which is a form of oppression.

Heath [223] argues that in collaborative dialogue, stakeholders negotiate power from a position of mutual interest. Heath argues further that community collaboration is better achieved through dialogue among the stakeholders and that emphasises creative outcomes in the communication. Heath exemplifies the diversity in ideas leading to innovation and creativity through negotiation of power and reciprocity in relationships. Heath found that the reciprocity and symmetry visible during the conversations encourage further dialogue among the stakeholders to develop a shared understanding. Heath sees dialogic moments as the means of transformation to gain community collaboration.

So, Freire [221], Young [136] and Heath [223] see oppression as the central issue of current society. I support their perspectives of understanding oppression and the theoretical approach of critical feminism which focuses on fighting against oppression for social equality. Using these frameworks provide the opportunity to act for liberation through ending oppression in society. The concept of oppression, mediation, collaboration and liberation is consistent with the key arguments of critical feminism which values the collective ownerships and shared understanding of childbirth experiences of women. Consistent with the socio-cultural perspective of childbirth, critical feminism offers opportunity to acknowledge women as the expert of their experiences and give power to them to decide about where and how they like to experience their birth. I argue that this is the only way women can take control of the place, process and experiences while giving birth without compromising their sense of safety.

Childbirth in remote Himalayas: a complex reality

The Western biomedical approach to childbirth considers the birth as an individual experience, and so, broader contexts beyond the individual are outside of the scope of this approach [71]. This model does not consider a broader community environment and disregards the notion of collective ownerships of experiences [224]. The biomedical approach is limited in understanding the experiences of rural women of Nepal where more than 90% of births happen outside the medical setting, with the support of family members, TBAs and other female relatives [31]. The socio-cultural approach is the best way to understand, analyse and make the meaning of childbirth experiences of women living in remote mountain villages of Nepal.

The Nepalese government aims to reduce medical risks during pregnancy, childbirth and postnatal period. The overall goal of the safe motherhood plan of the government is to improve maternal and neonatal survival especially among poor and socially excluded communities [10]. The government's safe motherhood plan focuses on changing the practices of the people to increase the utilisation of emergency obstetric care services where an increased emphasis is given to attend the birth by an SBA (doctors, nurses and assistant nurse midwives), birth preparedness and the readiness for complications [6]. This plan is informed by biomedical evidence, and the approach that the government has taken is focused on increasing institutional birth to reduce maternal and newborn mortality [2]. Although it is important to ensure that each woman has access to care, the government has not taken consideration of broader social factors impacting childbirth in remote areas of the country.

The medical assumption of averting childbirth risks through continued surveillance and medical interventions do not really work in the context of women in the mountains who follow traditions and cultural beliefs for their safety. Nepalese society is mostly collectivist in nature and childbirth is a culturally enriching experience. This leads to women's preference for giving birth in the community which gives them the opportunity to involve family members and other trusted support persons to control the birth process [1]. This notion of control is significant to women and family to continue the childbirth tradition. In the medical setting where the birthing process is controlled by professionals, it does not give any authority to women or their family members to have a say. This is not what the women or a family living in rural and remote areas of Nepal prefer to see, rather they prefer to stay at home to give birth.

There is an increasing attempt to promote institutional birthing practice in Nepal [225–227]. The Government of Nepal has introduced cash incentives to women if they attend antenatal checks and have an institutional birth [10, 228–230]. There are other funds offered at the community level for women and families accessing medical services during pregnancy and childbirth [191]. The incentive schemes and other funds related to increased utilisation of services are good attempts to do this; however, using it as a motivating factor limits the ability of women to make choices according to their preferences. The healthcare system is trying to force women to follow the medical model of pregnancy and childbirth with the incentive strategies. Nevertheless, women are not keen to go to hospital and prefer continuing the traditional practice [2].

Although it is important to address the higher maternal and neonatal mortality rates, the medicalisation of birth raises serious concerns for women in relation to their ability to make choices about the birth [231]. I took the opportunity to gather childbirth stories of women living in remote mountain villages in Nepal, and it was enlightening to go through their insightful childbirth experiences filled with significant culture, spirituality and tradition. It enabled me to understand their sense of safety while continuing the traditions and cultural practice.

Culture, tradition, religion and spirituality are significant to South Asian women when it comes to childbirth, and it is important to acknowledge this while understanding their stories. Giving opportunity to women, their family members and other significant people from the community to share their experiences could be one step towards understanding what is happening in relation to childbirth in mountain villages. It is also important to recognise many forces which oppress women within their community. As intended, this understanding enables the way to make childbirth a liberating experience to women.

Amidst this growing concern there remains a limited understanding of childbirth experiences of women living in remote mountain areas and how appropriate the institutional birth could be for them. Evidence is limited from urban and semi-urban areas where remote areas share completely different contexts in terms of demographic, socio-economic and geographic sense. The stories captured and shared in this book will provide insights to those dimensions and how that relates to the childbirth experiences of women.

Conclusion

Childbirth is a culturally and socially significant experience for women around the world. In some cultures, childbirth is a ritually polluted event and symbolises a rich tradition that women are expected to follow for their safety. Given the rise of the medical control of birth based on the notion of risks, women tend to lose ownership of their own birthing experiences. Evidence suggests that when women are unable to practice the tradition, their perception of safety is threatened. The socio-cultural perspective of childbirth has historically critiqued the medical model for making women powerless to decide how they would like to experience the birth.

Taking a socio-cultural lens, I argued that women should have choices to make their childbirth a safe, satisfying and empowering experience. I position the argument with the support of evidence from theories and research to contextualise the childbirth experiences of women in the remote mountains. With the commitment to value traditional knowledge, cultural practices and social values, I justify the need of taking socio-cultural view to understand the meaning of childbirth in a complex context of living. Acknowledging the impacts of broader social and structural determinants in health, I discuss how the differences in childbirth outcomes can be addressed to promote maternal and newborn survival in resource limited settings.

The critical feminist and social constructionist approaches are chosen to be the most authentic and relevant frameworks to examine the experiences of women within the circumstances of their childbirth. The evidence and arguments provided in this chapter will be referred consistently for the subsequent discussions to analyse the childbirth experiences of women in the remote mountains. Using lived experiences of women, more arguments will be formed to emphasise the place of traditional knowledge and cultural safety within the social construct of childbirth.

References

1   Basnyat, I., *Beyond biomedicine: Health through social and cultural understanding.* Nursing Inquiry, 2011. **18**(2): p. 123–134.
2   Kaphle, S., H. Hancock, and L.A. Newman, *Childbirth traditions and cultural perceptions of safety in Nepal: Critical spaces to ensure the survival of mothers and newborns in remote mountain villages.* Midwifery, 2013. **29**(10): p. 1173–1181.
3   Lupton, D., *Medicine as culture: Illness, disease and the body in western societies.* 2003: Sage Publications, Thousand Oaks.

4   Teman, E., *Childbirth, midwifery and concepts of time – Edited by Christine McCourt; foreword: Ronnie Frankenberg*. Journal of the Royal Anthropological Institute, 2011. **17**(1): p. 196–197.

5   Regmi, K. *Childbirth practices in Nepal: A review of models for reducing adverse outcomes*. International Journal of Gynaecology and Obstetrics, 2009. **107**(2): p. 321.

6   Kaphle, S., *Uncovering the covered: Pregnancy and childbirth experiences of women living in remote mountain areas of Nepal*. 2012: Flinders University, School of Medicine, Discipline of Public Health, Adelaide.

7   Douglas, V.K., *The Rankin Inlet birthing centre: Community midwifery in the Inuit context*. International Journal of Circumpolar Health, 2011. **70**(2): p. 178–185.

8   Lori, J.R. and J.S. Boyle, *Cultural childbirth practices, beliefs, and traditions in post conflict Liberia*. Health Care for Women International, 2011. **32**(6): p. 454–473.

9   Mann, J.R., et al., *Religion, spirituality, social support, and perceived stress in pregnant and postpartum Hispanic women*. Journal of Obstetric, Gynaecologic and Neonatal Nursing, 2010. **39**(6): p. 645–657.

10 Barker, C.E., et al., *Support to the safe motherhood programme in Nepal: An integrated approach*. Reproductive Health Matters, 2007. **15**(30): p. 81–90.

11 Walsh, D.J., *Childbirth embodiment: Problematic aspects of current understandings*. Sociology of Health and Illness, 2010. **32**(3): p. 486–501.

12 Oakley, A., *The captured womb: A history of the medical care of pregnant women*. 1984: Blackwell Publishing, Oxford.

13 Callister, L.C., S. Semenic, and J.C. Foster, *Cultural and spiritual meanings of childbirth: Orthodox Jewish and Mormon women*. Journal of Holistic Nursing, 1999. **17**(3): p. 280–295.

14 Steinberg, S., *Childbearing research: A transcultural review*. Social Science and Medicine, 1996. **43**(12): p. 1765–1784.

15 Regmi, K., R. Smart, and J. Kottler, *Understanding gender and power dynamics within the family: A qualitative study of Nepali women's experience*. Australian and New Zealand Journal of Family Therapy, 2010. **31**(2): p. 191–201.

16 Alp, K.Ö. and M. Özdemir, *The tradition of presenting gold gifts after giving birth in Anatolia*. Folk Life, 2010. **48**(1): p. 35–47.

17 Downe, S. and C. McCourt, *From being to becoming: Reconstructing childbirth*. Normal Childbirth E-Book: Evidence and Debate, 2008: Churchill Livingstone.

18 Heilemann, M.V., et al., *Acculturation and perinatal health outcomes among rural women of Mexican descent*. Research in Nursing and Health, 2000. **23**(2): p. 118–125.

19 Lewallen, L.P., *The importance of culture in childbearing*. Journal of Obstetric, Gynaecologic and Neonatal Nursing, 2011. **40**(1): p. 4–8.

20 Bolam, A., et al., *Factors affecting home delivery in the Kathmandu Valley, Nepal*. Health Policy and Planning, 1998. **13**(2): p. 152–158.

21 Homsy, J., et al., *Traditional health practitioners are key to scaling up comprehensive care for HIV/AIDS in sub-Saharan Africa*. Aids, 2004. **18**(12): p. 1723–1725.

22 Kamal, I.T., *The traditional birth attendant: A reality and a challenge*. International Journal of Gynaecology and Obstetrics, 1998. **63**: p. S43–S52.

23 Lefeber, Y. and H.W. Voorhoeve, *Indigenous customs in childbirth and childcare*. 1998: Uitgeverij Van Gorcum, Assen.

24 Mesko, N., et al., *Care for perinatal illness in rural Nepal: A descriptive study with cross-sectional and qualitative components*. BMC International Health and Human Rights, 2003. **3**(1): p. 3.

25 Lupton, D., *Medicine as culture: Illness, disease and the body*. 2012: Sage Publications, Thousand Oaks.

26 Kontos, N., *Perspective: Biomedicine – menace or straw man? Re-examining the biopsychosocial argument*. Academic Medicine, 2011. **86**(4): p. 509–515.

27 Bryers, H.M. and E. Van Teijlingen, *Risk, theory, social and medical models: A critical analysis of the concept of risk in maternity care*. Midwifery, 2010. **26**(5): p. 488–496.

28 Sargent, C. and L. Gulbas, *Situating birth in the anthropology of reproduction*. A Companion to Medical Anthropology, 2011. **10**(e037932): p. 289–303.

29 Thapa, S., *Challenges to improving maternal health in rural Nepal*. The Lancet, 1996. **347**(9010): p. 1244–1246.

30 Brunson, J., *Confronting maternal mortality, controlling birth in Nepal: The gendered politics of receiving biomedical care at birth*. Social Science and Medicine, 2010. **71**(10): p. 1719–1727.

31 Bennett, L., D.R. Dahal, and P. Govindasamy, *Caste, ethnic, and regional identity in Nepal: Further analysis of the 2006 Nepal Demographic and Health Survey*. 2008: Ministry of Health and Population, Government of Nepal, Kathmandu.

32 Thapa, N., et al., *Infant death rates and animal-shed delivery in remote rural areas of Nepal*. Social Science and Medicine, 2000. **51**(10): p. 1447–1456.

33 Dahal, K., *Nepalese woman dies after banishment to shed during menstruation*. British Medical Journal, 2008. **337**: p. a2520.

34 Schubert, J., G. Pillai, and R. Thorndahl, *Breaking the mold: Expanding options for reproductive health awareness: The CARE experience*. Advances in Contraception, 1997. **13**(2–3): p. 355–361.

35 Henderson, J., *Expert and lay knowledge: A sociological perspective*. Nutrition and Dietetics, 2010. **1**(67): p. 4–5.

36 Popay, J., et al., *Theorising inequalities in health: The place of lay knowledge*. Sociology of Health and Illness, 1998. **20**(5): p. 619–644.

37 Raymond, C.M., et al., *Integrating local and scientific knowledge for environmental management*. Journal of Environmental Management, 2010. **91**(8): p. 1766–1777.

38 Popay, J. and G. Williams, *Public health research and lay knowledge*. Social Science and Medicine, 1996. **42**(5): p. 759–768.

39 Lozoff, B., B. Jordan, and S. Malone, *Childbirth in cross-cultural perspective*. Marriage and Family Review, 1988. **12**(3–4): p. 35–60.

40 Newton, N. and M. Mead, Pregnancy, childbirth, and outcome: A review of patterns of culture and future research needs, in *Childbearing-Its Social and Psychological Aspects*. 1967: Williams and Wilkins, Baltimore.

41 Oakley, A., *Becoming a mother*. 1979: Schocken, New York.

42 Kitzinger, S., *Some cultural perspectives of birth*. British Journal of Midwifery, 2000. **8**(12): p. 746–750.

43 Smith, S.L. and S. Neupane, *Factors in health initiative success: Learning from Nepal's newborn survival initiative*. Social Science and Medicine, 2011. **72**(4): p. 568–575.

44 Diener, E., Introduction – Culture and well-being works by Ed Diener, in *Culture and well-being*. 2009: Springer. p. 1–8.

45 Rozario, S. and G. Samuel, *Daughters of Hariti: Childbirth and female healers in South and Southeast Asia*. 2003: Routledge, London.

46 Adhikari, R., *Demographic, socio-economic, and cultural factors affecting fertility differentials in Nepal*. BMC Pregnancy and Childbirth, 2010. **10**(1): p. 19.

47 Adhikari, R. and Y. Sawangdee, *Influence of women's autonomy on infant mortality in Nepal*. Reproductive Health, 2011. **8**(1): p. 7.

48 Karas, D.J., et al., *Home care practices for newborns in rural southern Nepal during the first 2 weeks of life.* Journal of Tropical Paediatrics, 2012. **58**(3): p. 200–207.

49 Shrestha, B.P., et al., *Community interventions to reduce child mortality in Dhanusha, Nepal: Study protocol for a cluster randomized controlled trial.* Trials, 2011. **12**(1): p. 1–14.

50 Stone, L., *Primary health care for whom? Village perspectives from Nepal.* Social Science and Medicine, 1986. **22**(3): p. 293–302.

51 Osrin, D., et al., *Cross sectional, community based study of care of newborn infants in Nepal.* British Medical Journal, 2002. **325**(7372): p. 1063.

52 Davis-Floyd, R., *The technocratic, humanistic, and holistic paradigms of childbirth.* International Journal of Gynaecology and Obstetrics, 2001. **75**(1): p. 5–23.

53 Davis-Floyd, R.E., *Birth as an American rite of passage: With a new preface.* 2004: University of California Press, Oakland.

54 Davis-Floyd, R.E. and C.F. Sargent, *Childbirth and authoritative knowledge: Cross-cultural perspectives.* 1997: University of California Press, Oakland.

55 Levesque, L.T., *Being pregnant: There is more to childbirth than having a baby.* 1980: Diliton, Ontario.

56 Records, K. and B.L. Wilson, *Reflections on meeting women's childbirth expectations.* Journal of Obstetric, Gynaecologic and Neonatal Nursing, 2011. **40**(4): p. 394–398.

57 Stevens, T., *Power and professionalism in midwifery practice: Impediment or precursor to normal birth.* Promoting Normal Birth: Research, Reflections and Guidelines. 2011: Fresh Heart Publishing, Durham. p. 150–159.

58 Carlo, W.A., et al., *High mortality rates for very low birth weight infants in developing countries despite training.* Paediatrics, 2010. **126**(5): p. 1072–1080.

59 Carlough, M., *More than hospitals are needed in Nepal.* Safe Motherhood, 1997(24): p. 9.

60 Johanson, R., M. Newburn, and A. Macfarlane, *Has the medicalisation of childbirth gone too far?* British Medical Journal, 2002. **324**(7342): p. 892–895.

61 Riessman, C.K., *Women and medicalization: A new perspective.* Social Policy, 1992. **14**(1): p. 3–18.

62 Souza, J.P., et al., *An emerging "maternal near-miss syndrome": Narratives of women who almost died during pregnancy and childbirth.* Birth, 2009. **36**(2): p. 149–158.

63 Hadjigeorgiou, E., et al., *Women's perceptions of their right to choose the place of childbirth: An integrative review.* Midwifery, 2012. **28**(3): p. 380–390.

64 Kitzinger, S., *Rediscovering birth.* 2011: Pinter and Martin Publishers, Chester.

65 Kitzinger, S., *Birth your way – Choosing birth at home or in a birth centre. A guide for pregnant women.* 2011: Fresh Heart Publishing, Chester.

66 Lupton, D. and J. Tulloch, *Risk is part of your life': Risk epistemologies among a group of Australians.* Sociology, 2002. **36**(2): p. 317–334.

67 Van Teijlingen, E., P. Simkhada, and J. Stephens, *We are all to blame!* Republica, 2010. **22**.

68 Reiger, K., *Our Bodies our babies: The forgotten women's movement.* 2001: Melbourne University Publishing, Melbourne.

69 Gunew, S., Feminist knowledge: Critique and construct, in *Feminist knowledge: Critique and construct.* 1990: Routledge, London.

70 Gunew, S.M., *A reader in feminist knowledge.* 1991: Routledge, London.

71 Conrad, P. and K.K. Barker, *The social construction of illness: Key insights and policy implications.* Journal of Health and Social Behavior, 2010. **51**(1): p. S67–S79.

72 Oswald, I., *Are traditional healers the solution to the failures of primary health care in rural Nepal?* Social Science and Medicine, 1983. **17**(5): p. 255–257.

73   Weingarten, K., *The discourses of intimacy: Adding a social constructionist and feminist view.* Family Process, 1991. **30**(3): p. 285–305.

74   Davis, D.L. and K. Walker, *Re-discovering the material body in midwifery through an exploration of theories of embodiment.* Midwifery, 2010. **26**(4): p. 457–462.

75   Jordan, B., *Birth in four cultures: A cross-cultural investigation of childbirth in Yucatan, Holland, Sweden and the United States.* 1978: Waveland Press, Long Grove.

76   Douglas, M., *Purity and danger: An analysis of concepts of pollution and taboo.* 2003: Routledge, London.

77   Douglas, V., *Childbirth among the Canadian Inuit: A review of the clinical and cultural literature.* International Journal of Circumpolar Health, 2006. **65**(2): p. 117–132.

78   Callister, L.C. and I. Khalaf, *Culturally diverse women giving birth: Their stories*, in *Childbirth across cultures.* 2009: Springer, New York. p. 33–39.

79   Callister, L.C. and I. Khalaf, *Spirituality in childbearing women.* The Journal of Perinatal Education, 2010. **19**(2): p. 16–24.

80   Callister, L.C., S. Semenic, and J.C. Foster, *Cultural and spiritual meanings of childbirth: Orthodox Jewish and Mormon women.* Journal of Holistic Nursing, 1999. **17**(3): p. 280–295.

81   Downe, S., et al., *What matters to women during childbirth: A systematic qualitative review.* PloS One, 2018. **13**(4).

82   Markens, S., C.H. Browner, and H. Mabel Preloran, *Interrogating the dynamics between power, knowledge and pregnant bodies in amniocentesis decision making.* Sociology of Health and Illness, 2010. **32**(1): p. 37–56.

83   Crotty, M., *The foundations of social research: Meaning and perspective in the research process.* 1998: Sage Publications, Thousand Oaks.

84   Downe, S., K. Finlayson, and A. Fleming, *Creating a collaborative culture in maternity care.* Journal of Midwifery and Women's Health, 2010. **55**(3): p. 250–254.

85   Kitzinger, S., *Authoritative touch in childbirth: A cross-cultural approach.* 1997: University of California Press, Berkeley.

86   Oakley, A., *Childbirth practice should take women's wishes into account.* BMJ: British Medical Journal, 1996. **313**(7071): p. 1557.

87   Hodnett, E.D., S. Downe, and D. Walsh, *Alternative versus conventional institutional settings for birth.* Cochrane Database of Systematic Reviews, 2012(8).

88   Hodnett, E.D., et al., *Continuous support for women during childbirth.* Cochrane Database of Systematic Reviews, 2013(7).

89   Boucher, D., et al., *Staying home to give birth: Why women in the United States choose home birth.* Journal of Midwifery and Women's Health, 2009. **54**(2): p. 119–126.

90   Olsen, O., *Promoting home birth in accordance with the best scientific evidence.* Promoting Normal Birth: Research, Reflections and Guidelines. 2011: Fresh Heart Publishing, Chester. p. 80–87.

91   Rijnders, M.E.B., *Interventions in midwife led care in the Netherlands to achieve optimal birth outcomes: Effects and women's experiences.* 2011: Universiteit van Amsterdam [Host], Amsterdam.

92   Rothman, B.K., *Recreating motherhood.* 2000: Rutgers University Press, New Brunswick.

93   Acharya, P.P. and D. Rimal, Pregnancy and childbirth in Nepal: Women's role and decision-making power, in *Childbirth across cultures.* 2009: Springer, New York. p. 137–144.

94   Benson, J., et al., *The impact of culture and ethnicity on women's perceived role in society and their attendant health beliefs.* InnovAiT, 2010. **3**(6): p. 358–365.

95 Morley, C. and S. Macfarlane, *The nexus between feminism and postmodernism: Still a central concern for critical social work*. British Journal of Social Work, 2012. **42**(4): p. 687–705.

96 Squire, C., *The social context of birth*. 2017: CRC Press, Boca Raton.

97 Mansfield, B., *The social nature of natural childbirth*. Social Science and Medicine, 2008. **66**(5): p. 1084–1094.

98 Hodnett, E., et al., *Continuous support for women during childbirth*. Birth, 2005. **32**(1): p. 72–72.

99 Callister, L.C., *Making meaning: Women's birth narratives*. Journal of Obstetric, Gynaecologic, and Neonatal Nursing, 2004. **33**(4): p. 508–518.

100 Douglas, M., *Risk and Blame: An analysis of concepts of pollution and taboo*. 1992: Routledge, London.

101 Callister, L.C., *Cultural meanings of childbirth*. Journal of Obstetric, Gynaecologic and Neonatal Nursing, 1995. **24**(4): p. 327–331.

102 Callister, L.C., K. Vehvilainen-Julkunen, and S. Lauri, *Cultural perceptions of childbirth: A cross-cultural comparison of childbearing women*. Journal of Holistic Nursing, 1996. **14**(1): p. 66–78.

103 Khalaf, I.A. and L.C. Callister, *Cultural meanings of childbirth: Muslim women living in Jordan*. Journal of Holistic Nursing, 1997. **15**(4): p. 373–388.

104 Sandall, J., C. Morton, and D. Bick, *Safety in childbirth and the three 'C's: Community, context and culture*. Midwifery, 2010. **26**(5): p. 481–482.

105 Smythe, E., *Safety is an interpretive act: A hermeneutic analysis of care in childbirth*. International Journal of Nursing Studies, 2010. **47**(12): p. 1474–1482.

106 Lupton, D., *Risk and sociocultural theory: New directions and perspectives*. 1999: Cambridge University Press, Cambridge.

107 Lupton, D., G. Mythen, and S. Walklate, *Beyond the risk society: Critical reflections on risk and human security*. 2006: Open University Press, Berkshire.

108 Eckermann, L., *Finding a 'safe' place on the risk continuum: A case study of pregnancy and birthing in Lao PDR*. Health Sociology Review, 2006. **15**(4): p. 374–386.

109 Kildea, S., et al., *Implementing birthing on country services for Aboriginal and Torres Strait Islander families: RISE framework*. Women and Birth, 2019. **32**(5): p. 466–475.

110 Kildea, S. and M. Wardaguga, Childbirth in Australia: Aboriginal and Torres Strait islander women, in *Childbirth across cultures*. 2009: Springer, New York. p. 275–286.

111 Kruske, S., S. Kildea, and L. Barclay, *Cultural safety and maternity care for Aboriginal and Torres Strait Islander Australians*. Women and Birth, 2006. **19**(3): p. 73–77.

112 Liamputtong, P., *Pregnancy, childbirth and traditional beliefs and practices in Chiang Mai, Northern Thailand*, in *Childbirth across cultures*. 2009: Springer, New York. p. 175–184.

113 Rumbold, A.R., et al., *Delivery of maternal health care in Indigenous primary care services: Baseline data for an ongoing quality improvement initiative*. BMC Pregnancy and Childbirth, 2011. **11**(1): p. 16.

114 Luttrell, C., S. Quiroz, and K. Bird, *Operationalising empowerment: A framework for an understanding of empowerment within SDC*. Paper commissioned by the Livelihoods for Equity desk (L4E) in the Swiss Agency for Development and Cooperation (SDC). 2007: Inter-Cooperation and Overseas Development Institute, Bern.

115 Giddens, A., *The constitution of society: Outline of the theory of structuration*. 1984: University of California Press, Oakland.

116 Lindgren, H.E., et al., *Perceptions of risk and risk management among 735 women who opted for a home birth*. Midwifery, 2010. **26**(2): p. 163–172.

117 Crossley, M.L., *Childbirth, complications and the illusion of 'choice': A case study.* Feminism and Psychology, 2007. **17**(4): p. 543–563.

118 Dowswell, T., et al., *Alternative versus standard packages of antenatal care for low-risk pregnancy.* Cochrane Database of Systematic Reviews, 2015(7).

119 Mayor, S., *More women at low risk of problems should have midwife led care, says King's Fund.* 2011: British Medical Journal Publishing Group.

120 Beck, U., *Risk society: Towards a new modernity.* 1992: Sage Publications, Thousand Oaks.

121 Adam, B., et al., *The risk society and beyond: Critical issues for social theory.* 2000: Sage Publications, Thousand Oaks.

122 Giddens, A., *Risk and responsibility.* 1999: Blackwell Publishing, Hoboken.

123 Douglas, M., *Purity and danger: An analysis of conception of body and pollution.* 1991: Routledge, London.

124 Douglas, M., *Risk and blame.* 2013: Routledge, London.

125 Douglas, M. and A. Wildavsky, *Risk and culture: An essay on the selection of technological and environmental dangers.* 1983: University of California Press, Oakland.

126 Marmot, M., *Social determinants of health inequalities.* The Lancet, 2005. **365**(9464): p. 1099–1104.

127 Marmot, M., et al., *Closing the gap in a generation: Health equity through action on the social determinants of health.* The Lancet, 2008. **372**(9650): p. 1661–1669.

128 Kuokkanen, L. and H. Leino-Kilpi, *Power and empowerment in nursing: Three theoretical approaches.* Journal of Advanced Nursing, 2000. **31**(1): p. 235–241.

129 Connell, R.W., *Gender and power: Society, the person and sexual politics.* 2013: John Wiley and Sons, Hoboken.

130 Rodin, J. and I.L. Janis, *The social power of health-care practitioners as agents of change.* Journal of Social Issues, 1979. **35**(1): p. 60–81.

131 Buchmann, W.F., *Adherence: A matter of self-efficacy and power.* Journal of Advanced Nursing, 1997. **26**(1): p. 132–137.

132 Foucault, M., *Power/knowledge: Selected interviews and other writings, 1972–1977.* 1980: Vintage, London.

133 Foucault, M., M. Morris, and P. Patton, *Michel Foucault power, truth, strategy.* 1979: Feral Publications, Port Townsend.

134 Martin, E., *The woman in the body: A cultural analysis of reproduction Milton Keynes.* 1989: Open University Press, Berkshire.

135 Young, I.M., *Justice and the politics of difference.* 2011: Princeton University Press, Princeton.

136 Young, I.M., *Five faces of oppression. Rethinking Power.* 2014: State University of New York Press, New York.

137 Solar, O. and A. Irwin, *Social determinants of health discussion paper 2 (policy and practice).* A conceptual framework for action on the social determinants of health. 2010: World Health Organization, Geneva.

138 Wallerstein, N., *Empowerment to reduce health disparities.* Scandinavian Journal of Public Health, 2002. **30**(59): p. 72–77.

139 Israel, B.A., et al., *Health education and community empowerment: Conceptualizing and measuring perceptions of individual, organizational, and community control.* Health Education Quarterly, 1994. **21**(2): p. 149–170.

140 Zimmerman, M.A. and J. Rappaport, *Citizen participation, perceived control, and psychological empowerment.* American Journal of Community Psychology, 1988. **16**(5): p. 725–750.

141 Van Olmen, J., et al., *Primary health care in the 21st century: Primary care providers and people's empowerment*. 2010: Blackwell Publishing, Hoboken.

142 Laverack, G. and R. Labonte, *A planning framework for community empowerment goals within health promotion*. Health Policy and Planning, 2000. **15**(3): p. 255–262.

143 Laverack, G., *Health promotion practice: Power and empowerment*. 2004: Sage Publications, Thousand Oaks.

144 Ulfsdottir, H., et al., *Like an empowering micro-home: A qualitative study of women's experience of giving birth in water*. Midwifery, 2018. **67**: p. 26–31.

145 Lindgren, H. and K. Erlandsson, *Women's experiences of empowerment in a planned home birth: A Swedish population-based study*. Birth, 2010. **37**(4): p. 309–317.

146 Schneider, D.A., *Beyond the baby: Women's narratives of childbirth, change and power*. 2009: Smith College School for Social Work, Northampton.

147 Lazarus, E., *What do women want? Issues of choice, control, and class in American pregnancy and childbirth*. Medical Anthropology Quarterly, 1997. **8**(1): p. 25–46.

148 Sapkota, S., et al., *In the Nepalese context, can a husband's attendance during childbirth help his wife feel more in control of labour?* BMC Pregnancy and Childbirth, 2012. **12**(1): p. 49.

149 Mumtaz, Z. and S. Salway, *Understanding gendered influences on women's reproductive health in Pakistan: Moving beyond the autonomy paradigm*. Social Science and Medicine, 2009. **68**(7): p. 1349–1356.

150 Simkhada, B., M.A. Porter, and E.R. Van Teijlingen, *The role of mothers-in-law in antenatal care decision-making in Nepal: A qualitative study*. BMC Pregnancy and Childbirth, 2010. **10**(1): p. 34.

151 Shroff, M.R., et al., *Does maternal autonomy influence feeding practices and infant growth in rural India?* Social science and medicine, 2011. **73**(3): p. 447–455.

152 Brunson, J., *Son preference in the context of fertility decline: Limits to new constructions of gender and kinship in Nepal*. Studies in Family Planning, 2010. **41**(2): p. 89–98.

153 Fivush, R., *Speaking silence: The social construction of silence in autobiographical and cultural narratives*. Memory, 2010. **18**(2): p. 88–98.

154 McNamee, S. and L. Shawver, *Therapy as social construction*, in *Furthering Talk*. 2004: Springer. p. 253–270.

155 Quek, K.M.-T., et al., *Gender equality during the transition to parenthood: A longitudinal study of dual-career couples in Singapore*. Journal of Social and Personal Relationships, 2011. **28**(7): p. 943–962.

156 Stoppard, J., *Understanding depression: Feminist social constructionist approaches*. 2014: Routledge, London.

157 World Health Organisation, *Closing the gap in a generation: Health equity through action on the social determinants of health*. 2008: World Health Organization, Geneva.

158 Walby, S., *Gender transformations*. 1997: Psychology Press, London.

159 Stanley, D. and M. Lopez-Garza, *Status of women in Nepal*. Comparative Studies of South Asia, Africa and the Middle East, 1982. **2**(2): p. 48–54.

160 Godha, D., D.R. Hotchkiss, and A.J. Gage, *Association between child marriage and reproductive health outcomes and service utilization: A multi-country study from South Asia*. Journal of Adolescent Health, 2013. **52**(5): p. 552–558.

161 Yeung, W.-J.J., S. Desai, and G.W. Jones, *Families in southeast and South Asia*. Annual Review of Sociology, 2018. **44**(1146): p. 469–495.

162 Kitzinger, S., *Ourselves as mothers: The universal experience of motherhood*. 1995: Addison Wesley Publishing Company, Boston.

163 Oakley, A., *Women confined: Towards a sociology of childbirth.* 1980: Schocken, New York.

164 Joseph, N., et al., *Incidence, correlates and outcomes of low birth weight – A one-year longitudinal study.* Indian Journal of Public Health Research and Development, 2011. **2**(1): p. 63–67.

165 Lansakara, N., S.J. Brown, and D. Gartland, *Birth outcomes, postpartum health and primary care contacts of immigrant mothers in an Australian nulliparous pregnancy cohort study.* Maternal and Child Health Journal, 2010. **14**(5): p. 807–816.

166 Luo, Z.-C., et al., *Birth outcomes in the Inuit-inhabited areas of Canada.* CMAJ, 2010. **182**(3): p. 235–242.

167 Luo, Z.-C., et al., *Neighborhood socioeconomic characteristics, birth outcomes and infant mortality among First Nations and non-First Nations in Manitoba, Canada.* The Open Women's Health Journal, 2010. **4**: p. 55.

168 Myers, H.F., *Ethnicity-and socio-economic status-related stresses in context: An integrative review and conceptual model.* Journal of Behavioral Medicine, 2009. **32**(1): p. 9–19.

169 Urquia, M.L., J.W. Frank, and R.H. Glazier, *From places to flows. International secondary migration and birth outcomes.* Social science and Medicine, 2010. **71**(9): p. 1620–1626.

170 Blumenshine, P., et al., *Socioeconomic disparities in adverse birth outcomes: A systematic review.* American Journal of Preventive Medicine, 2010. **39**(3): p. 263–272.

171 Janevic, T., D.A. Savitz, and M. Janevic, *Maternal education and adverse birth outcomes among immigrant women to the United States from Eastern Europe: A test of the healthy migrant hypothesis.* Social science and Medicine, 2011. **73**(3): p. 429–435.

172 Lisonkova, S., et al., *Birth outcomes among older mothers in rural versus urban areas: A residence-based approach.* The Journal of Rural Health, 2011. **27**(2): p. 211–219.

173 Rosenthal, L. and M. Lobel, *Explaining racial disparities in adverse birth outcomes: Unique sources of stress for Black American women.* Social Science and Medicine, 2011. **72**(6): p. 977–983.

174 Liu, N., et al., *Neighbourhood family income and adverse birth outcomes among singleton deliveries.* Journal of Obstetrics and Gynaecology Canada, 2010. **32**(11): p. 1042–1048.

175 De Brouwere, V., F. Richard, and S. Witter, *Access to maternal and perinatal health services: Lessons from successful and less successful examples of improving access to safe delivery and care of the newborn.* Tropical Medicine and International Health, 2010. **15**(8): p. 901–909.

176 Fotso, J.-C., et al., *What does access to maternal care mean among the urban poor? Factors associated with use of appropriate maternal health services in the slum settlements of Nairobi, Kenya.* Maternal and Child Health Journal, 2009. **13**(1): p. 130–137.

177 Joseph, K., et al., *Socioeconomic status and perinatal outcomes in a setting with universal access to essential health care services.* CMAJ, 2007. **177**(6): p. 583–590.

178 Sharma, S.K., Y. Sawangdee, and B. Sirirassamee, *Access to health: Women's status and utilization of maternal health services in Nepal.* Journal of Biosocial Science, 2007. **39**(5): p. 671.

179 Acharya, L.B. and J. Cleland, *Maternal and child health services in rural Nepal: Does access or quality matter more?* Health Policy and Planning, 2000. **15**(2): p. 223–229.

180 Dhakal, S., et al., *Skilled care at birth among rural women in Nepal: Practice and challenges.* Journal of Health, Population and Nutrition, 2011. **29**(4): p. 371.

181 Sreeramareddy, C.T., et al., *Home delivery and newborn care practices among urban women in western Nepal: A questionnaire survey.* BMC Pregnancy and Childbirth, 2006. **6**(1): p. 27.

182 Ahmed, M., et al., *Socio-cultural factors favoring home delivery in Afar pastoral community, northeast Ethiopia: A qualitative study.* Reproductive Health, 2019. **16**(1): p. 1–9.

183 Ahmed, S., et al., *Economic status, education and empowerment: Implications for maternal health service utilization in developing countries.* PloS One, 2010. **5**(6).

184 Desai, S. and S. Alva, *Maternal education and child health: Is there a strong causal relationship?* Demography, 1998. **35**(1): p. 71–81.

185 Elo, I.T., *Utilization of maternal health-care services in Peru: The role of women's education.* Health Transition Review, 1992. **2**(1): p. 49–69.

186 Kruk, M.E., M.R. Prescott, and S. Galea, *Equity of skilled birth attendant utilization in developing countries: Financing and policy determinants.* American Journal of Public Health, 2008. **98**(1): p. 142–147.

187 Raghupathy, S., *Education and the use of maternal health care in Thailand.* Social Science and Medicine, 1996. **43**(4): p. 459–471.

188 Bambra, C., et al., *Tackling the wider social determinants of health and health inequalities: Evidence from systematic reviews.* Journal of Epidemiology and Community Health, 2010. **64**(4): p. 284–291.

189 Bhandari, A., M. Gordon, and G. Shakya, *Reducing maternal mortality in Nepal.* BJOG: An International Journal of Obstetrics and Gynaecology, 2011. **118**(s2): p. 26–30.

190 Halim, N., A.K. Bohara, and X. Ruan, *Healthy mothers, healthy children: Does maternal demand for antenatal care matter for child health in Nepal?* Health Policy and Planning, 2011. **26**(3): p. 242–256.

191 Morrison, J., et al., *Utilization and management of maternal and child health funds in rural Nepal.* Community Development Journal, 2010. **45**(1): p. 75–89.

192 Drummond, P.D., et al., *Barriers to accessing health care services for West African refugee women living in Western Australia.* Health Care for Women International, 2011. **32**(3): p. 206–224.

193 Mueller, K.J., et al., *Health status and access to care among rural minorities.* Journal of Health Care for the Poor and Underserved, 1999. **10**(2): p. 230–249.

194 Culhane, J.F. and R.L. Goldenberg, *Racial disparities in preterm birth.* Seminars in Perinatology, 2011. **35**(4): p. 234–239.

195 Thaddeus, S. and R. Nangalia, *Perceptions matter: Barriers to treatment of postpartum hemorrhage.* Journal of Midwifery and Women's Health, 2004. **49**(4): p. 293–297.

196 Matsuyama, A. and K. Moji, *Perception of bleeding as a danger sign during pregnancy, delivery, and the postpartum period in rural Nepal.* Qualitative Health Research, 2008. **18**(2): p. 196–208.

197 Obermeyer, C.M., *Pluralism and pragmatism: Knowledge and practice of birth in Morocco.* Medical Anthropology Quarterly, 2000. **14**(2): p. 180–201.

198 Thapa, N., et al., *High-risk childbirth practices in remote Nepal and their determinants.* Women and Health, 2001. **31**(4): p. 83–97.

199 Falle, T.Y., et al., *Potential role of traditional birth attendants in neonatal healthcare in rural southern Nepal.* Journal of Health, Population, and Nutrition, 2009. **27**(1): p. 53.

200 Rhee, V., et al., *Maternal and birth attendant hand washing and neonatal mortality in southern Nepal.* Archives of Paediatrics and Adolescent Medicine, 2008. **162**(7): p. 603–608.

201 Thatte, N., et al., *Traditional birth attendants in rural Nepal: Knowledge, attitudes and practices about maternal and newborn health*. Global Public Health, 2009. **4**(6): p. 600–617.

202 World Health Organisation, *Trends in maternal mortality 2000 to 2017: Estimates by WHO, UNICEF*. UNFPA, World Bank Group and the United Nations Population Division. Geneva.

203 Filippi, V., et al., *Maternal health in poor countries: The broader context and a call for action*. The Lancet, 2006. **368**(9546): p. 1535–1541.

204 Dahlberg, M., et al., *Being perceived as 'a real woman' or following one's own convictions: A qualitative study to understand individual, family, and community influences on the place of childbirth in Busia, Kenya*. Culture, Health and Sexuality, 2015. **17**(3): p. 326–342.

205 Wagle, R.R., S. Sabroe, and B.B. Nielsen, *Socioeconomic and physical distance to the maternity hospital as predictors for place of delivery: An observation study from Nepal*. BMC Pregnancy and Childbirth, 2004. **4**(1): p. 8–18.

206 Wardlaw, M., *Religion, emotion, and spirituality in American hospital childbirth*. Doctoral Dissertation, 2016: The University of Texas, Austin.

207 Hickey, S., et al., *The Indigenous birthing in an urban setting study: The IBUS study*. BMC Pregnancy and Childbirth, 2018. **18**(1): p. 431.

208 Adams, K., et al., *Challenging the colonisation of birth: Koori women's birthing knowledge and practice*. Women and Birth, 2018. **31**(2): p. 81–88.

209 Edson, G., *Shamanism: A cross-cultural study of beliefs and practices*. 2009: McFarland, Jefferson.

210 Ghimire, K. and R.R. Bastakoti, *Ethnomedicinal knowledge and healthcare practices among the Tharus of Nawalparasi district in central Nepal*. Forest Ecology and Management, 2009. **257**(10): p. 2066–2072.

211 Uprety, M. and S. Adhikary, *Perceptions and practices of society towards single women in the context of Nepal*. Occasional Papers in Sociology and Anthropology, 2009. **11**: p. 244–254.

212 Kohrt, B.A. and D.J. Hruschka, *Nepali concepts of psychological trauma: The role of idioms of distress, ethnopsychology and ethnophysiology in alleviating suffering and preventing stigma*. Culture, Medicine and Psychiatry, 2010. **34**(2): p. 322–352.

213 Eigner, D., *Social and cultural dynamics of traditional healing*. 2010: The National Defence Academy, Vienna.

214 Kunwar, R.M., K.P. Shrestha, and R.W. Bussmann, *Traditional herbal medicine in Far-west Nepal: A pharmacological appraisal*. Journal of Ethnobiology and Ethnomedicine, 2010. **6**(1): p. 35.

215 Luitel, S., *The social world of Nepalese women*. Occasional Papers in Sociology and Anthropology, 2001. **7**: p. 101–114. https://doi.org/10.3126/opsa.v7i0.1113

216 Bennett, L., *Gender, caste and ethnic exclusion in Nepal: Following the policy process from analysis to action*. 2005: The World Bank, Washington, DC.

217 Nast, H., *Women in the field: Critical feminist methodologies and theoretical perspectives*. Professional Geographer, 1994. **46**(1): p. 54–66.

218 Ironside, P.M., *Creating a research base for nursing education: An interpretive review of conventional, critical, feminist, postmodern, and phenomenological pedagogies*. Advances in Nursing Science, 2001. **23**(3): p. 72–87.

219 Hughes, K.P., *Feminist pedagogy and feminist epistemology: An overview*. International Journal of Lifelong Education, 1995. **14**(3): p. 214–230.

220 Kushner, K.E. and R. Morrow, *Grounded theory, feminist theory, critical theory: Toward theoretical triangulation*. Advances in Nursing Science, 2003. **26**(1): p. 30–43.

221 Freire, P., *Pedagogy of the oppressed*. 2018: Bloomsbury Publishing, New York.

222 Shor, I. and P. Freire, *A pedagogy for liberation: Dialogues on transforming education*. 1987: Greenwood Publishing Group, Westport.

223 Heath, R.G., *Rethinking community collaboration through a dialogic lens: Creativity, democracy, and diversity in community organizing*. Management Communication Quarterly, 2007. **21**(2): p. 145–171.

224 Torsvik, M. and M. Hedlund, *Cultural encounters in reflective dialogue about nursing care: A qualitative study*. Journal of Advanced Nursing, 2008. **63**(4): p. 389–396.

225 Borghi, J., et al., *Financial implications of skilled attendance at delivery in Nepal*. Tropical Medicine and International Health, 2006. **11**(2): p. 228–237.

226 Manandhar, M., *Ethnographic perspectives on obstetric health issues in Nepal: A literature review*. 2000: Options, London.

227 Mullany, L.C., et al., *Risk factors for umbilical cord infection among newborn of southern Nepal*. American Journal of Epidemiology, 2007. **165**(2): p. 203–211.

228 Ensor, T., S. Clapham, and D.P. Prasai, *What drives health policy formulation: Insights from the Nepal maternity incentive scheme?* Health Policy, 2009. **90**(2–3): p. 247–253.

229 Powell-Jackson, T. and K. Hanson, *Financial incentives for maternal health: Impact of a national programme in Nepal*. Journal of Health Economics, 2012. **31**(1): p. 271–284.

230 Powell-Jackson, T., et al., *The experiences of districts in implementing a national incentive programme to promote safe delivery in Nepal*. BMC Health Services Research, 2009. **9**(1): p. 97.

231 Fox, B. and D. Worts, *Revisiting the critique of medicalized childbirth: A contribution to the sociology of birth*. Gender and Society, 1999. **13**(3): p. 326–346.

3 Childbirth research in complex social settings
Methodological reflections

Introduction

It was about midnight on a December night in a remote district hospital of Humla. The snow was starting to fall. I was about to fall asleep in a tiny room adjacent to the hospital after preparing for a stakeholders' workshop scheduled for the next morning. I heard a knock on the door and opened it. It was the physician responsible for running services in the hospital. He said, "Madam, there is a woman brought to the hospital with severe bleeding. She is only 24 weeks pregnant and I don't know what to do. She came from a village about seven hours walk away." He paused, standing still at the door. I felt his rising stress and panic.

I was an experienced midwife at that time, but we did not have a blood transfusion or caesarean facility at the hospital. I went with him to see the woman – she was almost unconscious. We gave her a few injections to control the bleeding, but they did not help. The snow began falling more heavily and the expectant mother started getting weaker. The next morning, the heartbeat of her unborn baby stopped and flights to the district halted due to the heavy snowfall. Two hours later, the mother died. This tragic event was the catalyst for me to commence research into these complex cross-cultural settings to understand the realities better, so that lives could be saved. I sought to answer the question: what factors influence childbirth experiences of women living in remote mountain villages of Nepal?

Conducting research in a cross-cultural setting is a complex and challenging endeavour. Yet in my view, doing cross-cultural research is a rewarding and empowering experience for researchers. Methodological and theoretical issues in cross-cultural research have been extensively discussed in terms of design, ethics and the authenticity of data [1]. Some methodological challenges have been highlighted by other researchers conducting childbirth research in cross-cultural communities [2]. The importance of taking the socio-cultural context of participants into account while designing and conducting childbirth research has been a consistent focus of researchers [3–5]. I am providing methodological insights from my own experience of conducting research into childbirth experiences of women in a complex social setting of Nepal.

Research approach

There has been an ongoing debate around quantitative versus qualitative research approaches concerning the nature of scientific knowledge and the relationship to the phenomena of the study [6]. The biomedical research approach is limited in providing meaningful insights into people's experiences as it tends to favour the objective collection of data and ignores the stories, emotions, opinions, knowledge, perceptions and experiences of the people. Therefore, qualitative approaches are more suitable to conduct childbirth research in complex social settings [1–6].

Baum [7] identified four main applications of a qualitative approach: to study and explain the economic, political, social and cultural factors that influence health; to understand how people interpret health and disease and make sense of their health experience; to elaborate causal hypotheses emerging from epidemiological and clinical research; and to provide contextual data to improve the validity and cultural specificity of quantitative survey instruments. This coincides with Wilkinson [8] who argues that research should focus on identifying and understanding the influence of social determinants on health outcomes across the interdisciplinary boundaries they emerge from rather than just trying to understand what causes poor health outcomes. Smith [9] suggests researchers take an approach that allows research with people from complex social environments to be conducted in a respectful, ethical, sympathetic and useful way.

Feminist, social and cultural studies have a vested interest in understanding the context of people to explore how that influences the way they perceive and respond to different situations or phenomena. Anthropological and ethnographic research focus particularly on the culture that people live in and goes beyond words to make meaning of people's experiences which are an individually unique cultural construct.

As a novice researcher attempting to conduct a study of childbirth experiences in socially and culturally complex communities, I chose to take an approach that was flexible, adaptable and meaningful to the circumstances of women. I took Oakley's [10] argument on board that the rationale for studying what happens to women when they are giving birth is to explore why they react to childbirth in the way they do and how their experiences of childbirth can be enhanced. Taking a critical perspective, Oakley goes further in saying that "the complexities of childbirth experiences of women need an extensive sociological analysis of the relationships of experiences and birth outcomes" [11]. I can relate to this concept when it comes to analysing the socio-cultural circumstances of women going through their childbirth experiences, as it is often complex to understand while making meaning of childbirth as a unique collective experience.

A qualitative approach is more compatible with the central tenets of critical feminism, which allows women's voices to be heard, providing them with the opportunity to express their feelings, share their knowledge and explore their reality [12]. Although the complexity of understanding childbirth experiences of women has been discussed in the literature [13–15], there is limited evidence on ways of resolving these complex issues to ensure ownership of the knowledge and experiences of childbirth is taken by women. To address this issue, a social constructionist approach provides a grounding from which to research childbirth experiences which defines people's beliefs, interpretations of reality and resulting behaviours as socially constructed phenomena [16]. Using ethnography, critical feminism and a social constructionist approach to provide an epistemological basis for research allows us to explore the uniqueness and complexities of childbirth experiences in a culturally rich and collective society.

For research with women living in complex community structures and social systems, there is no one-size-fits-all approach. I recommend applying the various aspects of qualitative approaches that are relevant to the research phenomena and context of participants. For my research with women in remote mountain villages of Nepal, I could not adhere to a single approach, rather I applied different principles and approaches to make their childbirth a meaningful and authentic experience.

Methodological principles

I noted earlier that ethnography, social constructionism and critical feminism inform appropriate ways of deepening understandings of childbirth in complex community settings. With the aim of exploring the complexities, uniqueness and diversities of women's childbirth experiences, application of these approaches values community knowledge and gives authenticity to the sources from which such knowledge is constructed [17]. Departing from the notion of acknowledging community as expert in identifying problems and developing effective solutions [18], I followed three guiding principles to conduct childbirth research in complex social settings.

Experiences are an authentic source of knowledge

Feminist researchers emphasise the importance of valuing traditional knowledge while making meaning of childbirth experiences of women [19, 20]. I support the arguments that people within their context should be considered as experts while making meaning of their experiences. Popay and Williams [21, 22] posit a pivotal role for lay knowledge and suggest applying creative research methods so that this knowledge can be visible and accessible to everyone. In their view, knowledge is created through interactions between researchers and participants and that interactions contribute to producing new knowledge about experiences.

Van Manen [23] introduces the concept of relationality as a source of knowledge which is essential to women's experiences of giving birth. In my view, sources of knowledge surrounding childbirth emerge from the experiences that women go through and are passed down from one generation to another, mostly women to women. I argued earlier that the scientific basis of knowledge in the medical model of birth devalues the significance of personal knowing about childbirth. This contrasts with the approach in my research where women's traditional knowledge plays a crucial role.

Oakley [20] argued strongly that women's experiences of giving birth should be given higher credibility than the authoritative knowledge that controls birth and limits women's ability to personalise their experience. Childbirth is a lived experience in which women acquire knowledge about the phenomena, the process and the outcomes. This way of knowing helps women decide what actions they need to take, when and by whom, and how to make their experiences better. Listening to women share their lived experience, researchers validate the worth of that unique experience [24]. The following example from one of the participants in my research explains this viewpoint well.

> Rita is a primary school teacher. She has a two-year-old daughter. She was living in the town with her husband and daughter. Her husband had to go overseas for work. She is expecting a second child. Rita quit her job and went to the village to live with her in-laws. Though her daughter was born in hospital, she felt the need of her mother-in-law's support to give birth. She stopped going for prenatal check-ups and started following her mother-in-law's advice. Rita is confused about her decision but certain that the birth will go well in the experienced care of her mother-in-law.

Armstrong et al. [25] and Popay et al. [26] argue that people's personal accounts create meaning and incorporate the ways in which they interpret their reality, how this reality affects them and the way they think produces better outcomes. The example I shared above reflects how reality can shift the way that women trust and value knowledge for safe birth outcomes. The circumstances women are in often limit their options and that frames the experience to be more authentic and powerful. Macintyre [27] argues for giving importance to people's experiences in understanding social inequalities, including lay knowledge and their personal experiences in everyday life. In my research, I gave credibility to traditional knowledge and community supports by acknowledging that childbirth is both an individual and collective experience.

Experiences are naturally occurring interactions

Social research focuses on producing rich descriptions of social worlds congruent with how an individual interacts with or views it. Hammersley [16] describes this as a social interaction that can be subjected to empirical testing. There is enough evidence to confirm that acknowledging experiences as naturally occurring interactions allows researchers to respect the socio-cultural context of participants [28]. This concept in research seeks to understand social reality as it happens, which provides rich descriptions of interactions in natural settings [12]. Social researchers value naturally occurring interactions as authentic sources of information [29].

I valued this concept and adopted it as a guiding principle in my research. This allowed me to develop trust and familiarity with the research participants while interacting with them about their experiences of childbirth. It was important to me to respect the preferences of participants and what is accepted within their social environment rather than adhering to a structured research process. I kept interactions as fluid as possible in their everyday settings and documented them in multiple ways. In this way, interactions I had with participants were not only what they told me but also how and where those conversations occurred. Most interactions occurred during daily chores: cooking, washing, walking to the farm and carting water. The following scenario elicits why and how I had to respect the everyday life context and make meaning of experience as naturally occurring interactions.

> I sat in the corner of Thuli's house. Four other women came quickly and joined me. There was a 28-day-old baby on Thuli's lap wrapped in a dirty piece of towel. There were no clothes for the baby. The weather was cold. Thuli looked fragile and she could not hear me well. Initially I had no intuition as to where or how to start a conversation. Once I slowly started asking about her experience of giving birth, other women were quicker to answer than her. The setting became a group discussion rather than an interview. I listened to all conversations with equal respect and documented them. Yet, the emotional silence of Thuli was more powerful to me than the voices of the other women.

The whole scenario was worth being part of to understand and make meaning of it. I sensed the power imbalance between that mother and the other women in the village. Charon [30] argues that when an individual makes interpretations of their experiences, they link them both at individual and societal levels. In this process, personal experiences of childbirth become collective through the involvement of social interactions. Another scenario I encountered while interviewing a mother illustrates this further.

> I went to speak with a mother who had a baby at home. It was her 11th day. She was staying outside in a room at the corner of the house. Her father-in-law appeared at the front of the house as I was about to initiate interaction. Although I wanted to speak with the mother about her childbirth experience, the father-in-law insisted on being part of the conversation. I had to allow him to join in. The three of us were about 200 metres apart. Every time I prompted conversation; he was the one who answered while the mother said very little.

As childbirth is a part of everyday life events in remote mountain areas of Nepal, giving value to both individual and collective constructions of experiences as they occur in the participants' socio-cultural setting is pertinent. The two scenarios just presented confirm that it was critical for me to take all interactions into account while analysing women's childbirth experiences.

The researcher's reflexivity in research

The researcher's reflexivity is a key concept which determines the impact of the research process on the quality of research findings [23, 31–33]. Reflexivity is defined as a process of critical self-reflection and an acknowledgement of the inquirer's place in the setting, context and social phenomena he or she seeks to understand and is also a means for a critical examination of the entire research process [34]. Thus, the researcher's reflexivity represents a methodical process of learning about self as researcher, which, in turn, illuminates deeper, richer meanings about personal, theoretical, ethical and epistemological aspects of the research question [35]. Schwandt's [34] concept of reflexive process included in the definition refers to the documentation of the setting, context and phenomena.

Finlay and Gough [36] mentioned that reflexivity offers researchers ways to analyse how subjective and intersubjective elements influence their research. The use of reflexivity enables the transformation of subjectivity from a problematic issue into an opportunity; however, the process of engaging in reflexive analysis can be difficult for researchers [36, 37]. Finlay and Gough [36] outline the complexities of maintaining subjective and objective accounts in a reflexive engagement.

> Reflexivity taps into a more immediate, continuing, dynamic and subjective self-awareness. Having come to understand that the researcher, the world, and the researchers' experience of the world are intertwined, the challenge is to identify that lived experience that resides in the space between subject and object. The researcher strives to capture some of the connections by which subject and object influence and constitute each other.
>
> (p. 533)

Heidegger [38] argues that each person perceives the same situation differently, so it is vital to incorporate their own reflecting, intuiting and thinking to make meaning of data. Finlay [37] mentioned that social constructionists draw on the concept of reflexivity to explain how individuals make sense of the social world and their place in it. In this process, researchers are more outward focused into the realm of interactions, discourses and shared meanings. Social constructionists stress that reflexive analysis should take the dynamics of researcher-participant relationships into account to examine their impacts on research [35, 36, 39]. Van Manen [23] suggests using a "bracketing" approach in the reflexive analysis process, so the researcher can enter the lived experience and attend actively to the opinions of participants. This requires researchers to be aware of the factors or the context that needs to be bracketed.

My reflexivity in research was maintained through reflexive notes of each interview and reflexive journaling of my fieldwork. My role during fieldwork was to facilitate participants to share their experiences in relation to childbirth. I did that by helping them to talk about their perceptions, feelings, expectations, problems and experiences through in-depth interviewing. Despite my shared nationality, childbirth experience and language, I understood the difference between my position and the context of participants in the research. I bracketed them out, and it helped me to clear my pre-conceived understandings, assumptions, beliefs and judgements about the situation and the participants. I learnt these differences through reflexivity where bracketing remained a continuous process.

For example, the following note from my field journaling explains how reflexive analysis enabled me to clear pre-conceived assumptions.

> I am on my way to the fieldwork. I flew in from Kathmandu this morning. I am hoping to catch another flight to get to the mountain district tomorrow. This evening, I took the opportunity of having dinner with my former colleagues from UNICEF. Over dinner, we discussed the errors that development organizations are making in developing countries. We, as social scientists or development experts, use language that exploits the status of people. We called them "poor" ignoring the richness of their kindness, cultures and tradition. We called them "underprivileged" without acknowledging their strengths and rich potential. We try to exploit them with the tag of "poverty." Our language must change, and we should stop exploiting communities with power-laden terminology. They may not be poor or underprivileged. We should change the way we view them, how we define their status and how we conceptualize their life.

My reflexive analysis in this example demonstrates how I became aware of the language and categorisation by outsiders and decided not to think of my participants or the context of their community in that way. I had an opportunity to observe events and interactions happening within a family and the community in addition to having conversations with the participants. I documented these observations in reflexive journaling which gave me a better understanding of the family and their social circumstances. Another example from my field journaling demonstrates how reflexivity helped develop an understanding of the context of childbirth in remote villages.

> I was walking with a local man to reach Murma village. I saw a health post sign and went inside. There were two men sitting around the wood-fired oven. I introduced myself and learned that they were health workers. I explained my reason for going to Murma village and they told me that this village is the most backward and neglected one in the district. They mentioned to me that women in this village don't come for check-ups because they are shy. They think it is embarrassing to talk about pregnancy or childbirth. "You know, Sister, lots of babies died this year in that village. People are very conservative." One of them said. They were interested in continuing the conversation, but I thanked them for their insights and continued walking to the village.

This conversation helped me to understand how health workers described the context and situation of childbirth in the village. I noticed a victim-blaming approach and the use of language to frame the community and women as well. This reflexivity added value to the data as I analysed and interpreted the findings. Both my conversations with participants and engagement in conversations during field work combined with my observation of events enabled me to enhance the richness of the research data. I will provide further examples of how reflexivity was embedded throughout the research process in subsequent discussions.

The field work: crossing rivers and climbing mountains

Social science researchers discuss challenges and dilemmas concerning traditional ethics models which disregard more personal interactive and moral forms
of interaction in the fieldwork. The conditions of fieldwork that allow researchers
to form various types of relationships at personal and social levels are criticised in
terms of the moral and ethical dilemmas they pose to maintaining research standards [40–42]. Cross-cultural researchers argue that fieldwork enables research to
explore the everyday lives of people to gain understanding of their context and
the issues being examined [43–45]. In my view, fieldwork is the most exciting
and insightful part of research, where researchers not only collect data but also
learn other dimensions of the lives of people living in complex social settings.
This enables researchers to develop a deeper understanding of the phenomena of
their study by gaining trust of the community through sharing a complex social
environment and experiences.

For my research with women in Nepal, I conducted fieldwork in two remote
mountain villages. To uncover childbirth experiences of women in their everyday
life setting, I followed them in their daily activities inside and outside the home.
I wrote down my reflections every evening and included them in the field journaling. My reflections depicted my positionalities, which shifted according to the
situation or my dilemmas, as ethics protocols were challenged to accommodate
social expectations or my own complexities while living far away from family in
a remote community with no access to communication with the outside world or
basic resources.

On the day I reached Mugu village, I wrote:

> I left the district hospital this morning and walked 10 hours to reach Mugu
> village. I immersed myself in thought on the way. I crossed and recrossed the
> same river about seven times – sometimes on a bridge and sometimes hopping
> over rocks. I met a group of women reconstructing the path together. They
> were talking and laughing; it sounded like a fun time. They asked if I was
> a high school student! I started to ponder my status as a researcher from an
> Australian university, which didn't mean anything to these women. I saw don-
> keys carrying supplies, mostly rice, to the village. There were women carrying
> loads too. I climbed over five different mountains on the way. I couldn't imag-
> ine the women walking to the hospital to give birth; it seemed too hard. There
> were three tea stalls on the way, but I didn't stop for tea. I reached the village
> just below a snowy peak. The village was new to me and I was new to the vil-
> lagers. I started thinking about my daughter in Adelaide. Oh well, I can't even
> talk to her now. I saw many children, the same age as my daughter, playing
> outside. Watching them made me more aware of missing her. I said gently to
> myself, "I need to just wait and see what the morning brings . . .!"

Suwankhong and Liamputtong [42] provide a thick description of the positionality of the researcher while conducting fieldwork in a cross-cultural setting

regarding forming relationships with local people, learning new things to accommodate the social environment and gathering valuable socio-cultural insights. My experiences of conducting fieldwork in remote Nepal resonate with the reflections of other social science researchers who outlined similar complexities and moral-ethical dilemmas [40–42, 46, 47].

Given the climate and defined working seasons at high altitude in the mountains, I was in the field from February to May to avoid extreme weather conditions and heavy snowfall. Even during this period, it was still cold in the mountains. Families mostly sat and slept around the wood-fired oven in the kitchen to stay warm. They invited me to join in this setting in the house I shared during fieldwork. This gave me the opportunity to be part of conversations and observe what was happening in that environment. I felt fortunate to receive that level of acceptance, but at the same time it was not easy for me to adapt to the circumstances. I was not comfortable sharing a family space all the time but that was the respectful thing to do in the village.

There were no toilets in the village, and they gave me a key to the local health centre to use its toilet which was about a five-minute walk from the house. The nights were hard. There were no bathrooms or hot water for showers. I had to go to the public tap located in the middle of the village to bathe, which was open and mostly busy during the day. I chose to go to the tap before anyone was awake for a wash, the only suitable option. The water was usually freezing, and I walked there with a sense of fear. A woman came and asked, *"why do you need to bathe so frequently?"* and she said, *"in the village, we bathe once a month."* Yet, I was different to them. This behaviour reflected my position in the village, and it raised questions and confirmed differences. It shifted my position from an insider to an outsider and created an ethical dilemma.

Although I had never lived in this remote community, I felt I had a strong affiliation with the context and the research situation: as a mother, as a health professional who had worked in similar communities, as someone who could speak the same language, and as someone who had a similar social-cultural background, even though I was then living in another country. That is, I felt I would be able to take an "insider" perspective for my research. As such, I justified my ethics application based on this rationale. I have now spent a couple of days settling into the village, speaking with the local women, and finding my way around. The women made it quite clear to me that they did not feel I would be able to take an "insider" perspective because I was different. They noted that *"I am an educated woman who had an independent means of making a living, I dress and speak differently, I live in another country and as such I am a foreigner to them in their community."*

I was at first surprised at this suggestion and then started to feel very anxious about whether I would be able to continue my research without a formal review of my ethics approval to shift my positionality. I had based my methodology on taking the insider perspective. At the same time, I agreed with what the women were saying about the obvious differences between us as most of them had never been outside their village in their entire lives. It was true that they could not accept me as an "insider" with the limited bonds that we shared together. After discussing the situation with the Chair of the ethics committee based in Australia, we agreed that my position in the research would shift according to the situation and I would manage it to respect the choices participants make. Once the interactions started involving personal stories of childbirth, the women tended to say that *"we are similar but different."*

Other researchers have discussed a similar shift and the dilemmas of insider-outsider positions in cross-cultural research [41, 42, 45–49]. Despite these differences, I was able to establish a trusting relationship with the women through a shared identity, language and motherhood. All the women were delighted to welcome me into their homes, to share meals, to attend special events, to play with their children and to walk with them during their everyday chores.

This trusting relationship enabled open conversations about childbirth experiences which involved emotions of both happiness and trauma. It was a sensitive topic to discuss, especially with these women who had experienced multiple perinatal and neonatal losses. The trust women placed in me to share their experiences enabled me to manage these emotions effectively. We laughed and cried together. Women felt honoured to have the opportunity to speak.

One woman said, *"I don't know why you want me to tell my story. I am old and worthless. You want to learn about our times, which few want to know about these days. Even my children aren't interested in listening to me."* She started telling me about her experiences of childbirth and the traditions involved. It made them feel valued that I was there just to listen to their experiences when no one had done so before.

As soon as the snow started melting in April, the seasonal migration to the mountains to access high-altitude farming areas for growing potatoes and barley began. The family I was staying with needed to move as well. They suggested I stay back in the village with the young children and elderly people. I declined the offer and insisted on joining them and the other villagers in the high-altitude area for a week. We had to climb for several hours to reach the farmland. It was a totally different world, and it felt like a camping experience without the holiday atmosphere. I managed to continue interactions with many mothers, some of whom brought their infants with them, while some were expecting to give birth in couple of weeks. I became a babysitter and a helper to women. At the end of the day, the women had to cook for their families and the men mostly sat together, chatting and drinking traditional alcohol. It was another fascinating and eye-opening experience.

The field area

Many researchers emphasise the importance of the process of selecting a field area when conducting research into complex or sensitive issues in a cross-cultural community [40–47, 49, 50]. For my research, I purposely selected the most remote and disadvantaged area in the mountains of Nepal. I travelled from Adelaide to Kathmandu, the capital of Nepal. I had to take a further domestic flight to another town – Surkhet or Nepalgunj to reach this mountainous district. Mountain flights in Nepal are heavily dependent on weather conditions. For the first three days, I went to the local airport at 5:00 a.m., waited until midday and then returned to the hotel as flights were cancelled due to unfavourable weather. On the fourth day, I was finally able to fly.

With such uncertain flight conditions, people of political influence or of higher social status were given priority to secure seats. There were many local people who had been waiting for a week or more to fly home, as there was no other mode of transport to the mountains, were neglected. The flight was an interesting journey in and of itself as people kept asking why I had chosen such a difficult place to do this research. Amidst the challenges I experienced, I had a purpose and I remained committed.

I reflected on the challenges of the journey in my field notes.

> I was lucky to get a ticket for the local flight from Nepalgunj. On the first morning, I went to the airport at 5:30 a.m. (I was warned to go early) but the security guard did not let me in. He asked me to come back at 9 a.m. I went back to the hotel, returning to the airport gates at 9 a.m. Security told that the flight would leave at 1 pm and asked to come back around noon. Here we go, back to the hotel again. I was a little stressed about my schedule. What would happen if I could not fly today? It was about 11:30 a.m. when I rang the airline office. No one picked up the call. After half an hour, the travel agent called me and said the flight was about to leave. I packed everything and rushed to the airport. I checked in and waited outside with my boarding pass. After about an hour, an airline employee announced that the flight had been cancelled due to unfavourable weather conditions and please to return at 9 a.m. tomorrow.
>
> I needed to get my luggage back for the night. A member of the ground staff agreed to give it back to me and walked with me up to the gate. He asked, "which office do you come from, Madam"? I said, "I am a student." He conjectured, "you must be going to Rara lake." I told him the reason for my trip. He looked surprised and asked again; "why didn't you choose a place with easy access?" I replied, "because I want to understand the difficulties and hardships of people living in these remote areas. It is important to me to know how they manage their problems." He responded, "you are doing good work, Sister." We departed for the day.

Mugu is one of the poorest and most remote districts in Nepal [51]. Most families in Mugu only manage to grow enough food for six months of the year. The social structures, cultural practices and lifestyles of the people living in different parts of the district are diverse, reflecting various ethnic backgrounds. People living in the northern part of the district which bordered China are Indigenous groups and follow Tibetan customs and the Buddhist religion. These groups are known as the Lama people [52].

Only 5% of the total area of the Mugu district has fertile land which causes constant food insecurity. The average family size in the district is 6.1 where Chhetri

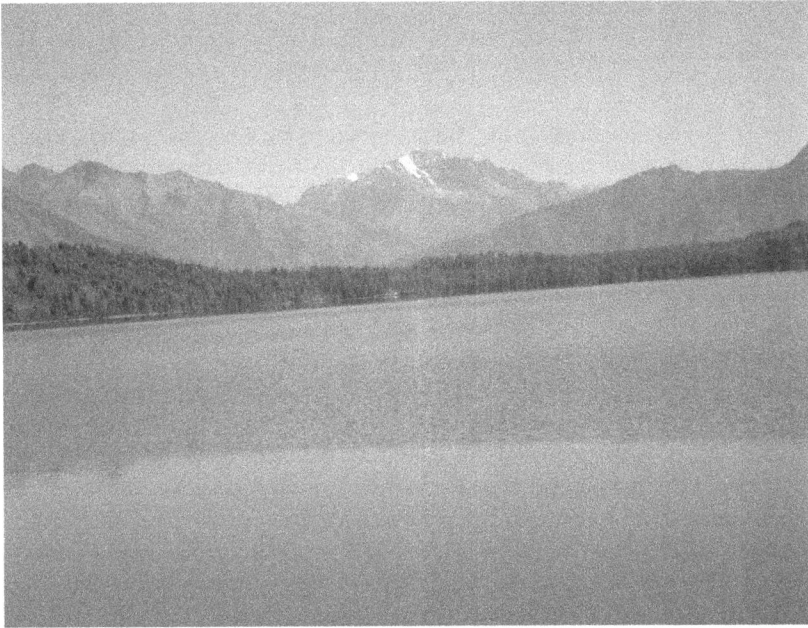

Figure 3.1 Geographic terrains of the Mugu district
Source: Picture taken by the author

is the predominant ethnicity (49%), followed by Indigenous Lama group (9%), with the remaining 42% of the population comprising numerous other ethnic groups [53]. Despite its beautiful landscape, challenges for people living in this district are critical.

Geographically, the district has distinct terrains. There is a beautiful lake located in the centre of the district called Rara. Different ethnic and cultural groups occupy the scattered villages across varied terrains. The district comprises different Village Development Committees, a local administrative unit of the Nepalese government. I conducted the research with a Chhetri group from Ruga village and a Lama group from Mugu village.

Within the Mugu district there are several health facilities at different levels of the health system: 1 district hospital, 1 Primary Health Care Centre (PHCC), 8 Health Posts (HP), 16 Sub Health Posts (SHP) and 2 Ayurvedic Health Care Centres (AHCC). At the time of research, only five of these health facilities, including the hospital, were providing maternal and newborn care services.

According to the district report, half of the population did not use the services provided in these health facilities because they were located at too great a distance, 7% expressed no trust in the care provided in these centres. A further 25% identified the problem of unavailability of health workers. More than 20% of people in the district preferred using traditional healers during illness rather than going to the healthcare centres.

Research villages

Chhetri village had comparatively better access to food because of their location being closer to district markets. They spoke the Nepali language and followed Hindu religion. Early marriage of girls was a common cultural practice in this village. Marriage in this group was usually arranged by parents according to their interests and preferences and occurred from 12 to 15 years of age. The duration of birth pollution in this village was 15–30 days. The Goth (cow shed) was the most common place of giving birth. This village had a birthing centre with a professionally trained midwife providing 24-hour services.

In Lama village, they used the Tibetan script in reading and writing and spoke Nepali to communicate with outsiders. The practice of early marriage was also common. Most of the marriages in this group occurred by negotiation between the girl and boy, and parents were not involved in that decision. Some women in this village gave birth in the Goth (cow shed) and others chose the outside corner of the house. The duration of childbirth pollution in this group varied from 3 to 15 days. They did not have any professional childbirth services available in the village; the closest medical help was at the district hospital.

Service initiatives and resources

Childbirth services and programmes in Nepal are based on the concept of "Safe Motherhood" introduced by the World Health Organisation and focus on family

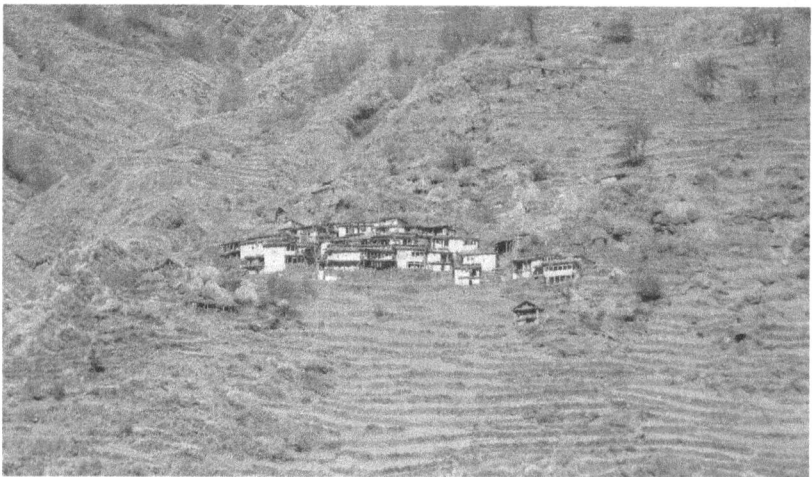

Figure 3.2 A research village located on the mountain of Nepal

Source: Picture taken by the author

planning, antenatal care, safe delivery and essential obstetric care [54]. The Government of Nepal launched the Nepal Safe Motherhood Project (NSMP) in March 1997 to improve maternal and neonatal survival and reduce related mortalities. The Government launched NSMP to only ten districts until 2004 and most of the remote districts were not included in the programme.

In 2005, the Department for International Development in the UK provided additional funding to implement the Maternal and Newborn Health Project (MNHP) through the Support to Safe Motherhood Programme in a few more districts of Nepal. Mugu, which was the lowest in the Human Development Index and had no emergency obstetric care services, was chosen for expansion of basic emergency obstetric care services in the district hospital and for the implementation of the MNHP in order to reduce maternal and newborn mortality. The United Mission to Nepal in partnership with the District Health Office (DHO) began implementation of the MNHP programme in Mugu from October 2005. This programme focused on service strengthening and community awareness raising, aiming to increase access to services and information. The district hospital started to provide 24-hour basic obstetric care in July 2006 and upgraded four health facilities located in four different areas to birthing centres to provide 24-hour services to women.

Since 2009, the national Government of Nepal has supported a safe birth incentive programme in which women were entitled to get 1500 rupees (approx. 20 USD)

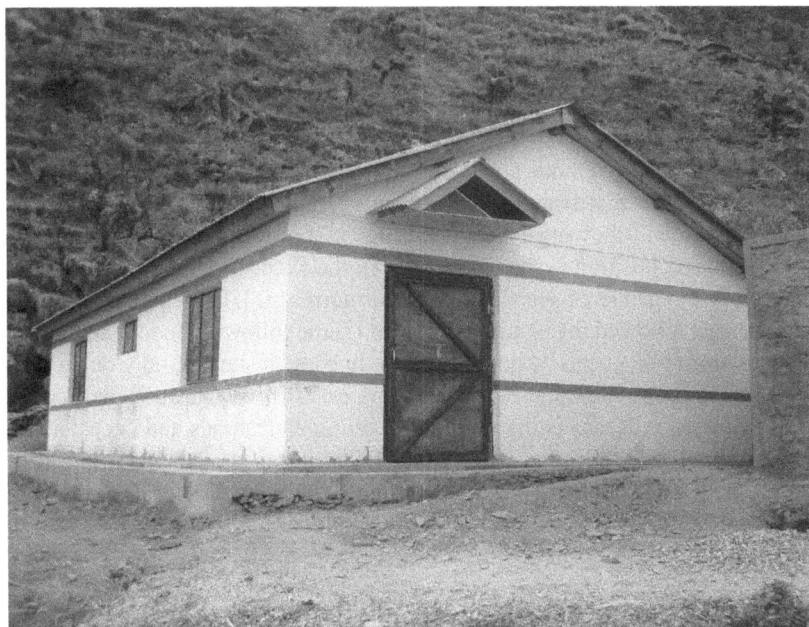

Figure 3.3 A birthing centre located halfway to the district hospital
Source: Picture taken by the author

if they gave birth in a district hospital or other certified birthing centre in mountain districts. The government also made provision for giving a cash incentive to women who make at least four visits during their pregnancy to a prenatal clinic. However, the impact of these initiatives on women's childbirth experiences was not effective in remote areas where services were geographically hard to access.

Women in remote mountain areas

A typical day for married women in remote mountain areas involves cleaning the house and fetching natural spring water before sunrise, making morning and evening tea and family meals, cleaning animal sheds twice daily and organising animal fodder, doing the dishes and laundry, attending private or communal farm work or tasks allocated to them, and wondering where to obtain food to feed their children and other family members. This becomes a daily routine which generally starts before 5:00 a.m. and ends around 9:00 pm with hardly any time left for themselves. Pregnancy and childbirth do not change the routine, and minimal attention or support is given by the family during pregnancy.

In Nepal, as in other developing countries, women are among the poorest and most vulnerable members of society. The situation of women living in the remote mountains of Nepal is different to women from other areas of the country because of their distinct socio-cultural patterns [55]. Most women in the remote mountainous areas are illiterate and not exposed to places beyond their social, geographical and physical boundaries [56]. The health status of women is low; they have a high burden of unpaid domestic and farm work, including the continuing burden of pregnancy, childbirth and childrearing [57]. At the time of research, women in Mugu had the lower life expectancy of 42 years compared with 44 years for men [58].

Women living in remote areas of Nepal are often known by outsiders as "oppressed" and "disadvantaged" because of their relative poverty [59, 60]. Although women following Tibetan and Buddhist philosophies have a comparatively respected position in their society [61], the status of Hindu women is marginalised due to gendered social and religious norms [55]. In the research villages, some women followed the Hindu religion and some followed Buddhism, but their practices were influenced by both religions. In some instances, only one of these philosophies drove their status and, in some cases, both did. In Nepal, cultural fusion between religions is the norm, with religious festivals and occasions celebrated equally by followers of different faiths. Even though according to the census in 2011, Hinduism is still the dominant religion in Nepal, all religious principles and constructs are blended in social practice.

Research process: participants, ethics and consent

There has been ongoing discussion that recruiting participants for involvement in a sensitive research topic could be challenging for researchers [62–64]. Researchers often try to fit into participant's lives and ask them to share their experiences which sometimes can be traumatic [4]. It is important that researchers are trained to manage such situations effectively while accessing the personal stories of participants for research purposes [46, 48]. Ethical and methodological dilemmas around informed consent, confidentiality, privacy, social justice and questions about power and contextual relevance while recruiting participants for sensitive research have been emphasised by many researchers [62–66]. I argue that recruiting participants from a complex social setting for involvement in a sensitive study requires the researcher to take their vulnerability into account, so that sharing their experiences does not result in negative consequences but provides a pathway to open about their grief, resentments and hopes for the future. This can be done by establishing a trusting relationship [4] and giving participants more power to share their story with the researcher [66].

For my research, the primary participants comprised either pregnant or postnatal women (given birth within four weeks prior to the interview date). Additionally, their husbands, their mothers-in-law and/or fathers-in-law, service providers and local stakeholders of the community were recruited to gather different perspectives. Using a standard strategy [67], a purposive sample of 25 pregnant or postnatal women were recruited using following criteria for an in-depth interview. Additionally, five husbands, five mothers-in-law and one father-in-law participated in an in-depth interview. Most husbands declined to participate saying childbirth is women's business and mentioned they have nothing to say. Interviews were conducted with five service providers and four local stakeholders directly involved in the childbirth care and decisions.

The recruitment process involved the use of local female community health volunteers (FCHVs) of the villages. In Nepal's health system, local FCHVs keep the record of pregnancies and childbirth in the village as they are the first point of contact for women. I met with the FCHVs to identify possible participants in the research. Then the FCHV approached these women for their willingness to be involved in research and collected interested women's names. Once confirmed, I approached all the women to arrange interviews. After I completed the interviews with the women, I approached their husbands, fathers-in-law and mothers-in-law for their willingness to participate. Finally, I identified service providers and local stakeholders in the community based on information revealed during the in-depth interviews with women and family members and invited them to participate in the study.

The complexities of gaining access to research participants for a qualitative study have been acknowledged in literature [44, 63]. Even though the use of local people who are often gatekeepers to potential study participants is accepted as one of the strategies of a qualitative study with the intention of minimising bias in participation [44], feminist researchers question this approach as it may result in significant pressure on women to be involved who are not in a social position to make decisions [68]. Keeping these complexities in mind, the use of the FCHV to recruit participants in this research was deemed appropriate.

Many qualitative researchers, and especially those working in critical approaches such as feminist research, have championed equality in the researcher and participant relationship. The status and integrity of research subjects are most visible now through mandatory ethical approval procedures [69]. The ethics approval process in this research was based on the concept of protection of individuals from harm through maintaining confidentiality, anonymity and informed consent. Qualitative researchers often take this further than a single approval process at the beginning of their studies by explicitly keeping participants informed at all stages of the research process, and by attempts to ensure that participants encounter respect, transparency and openness [70]. This emphasises an ethical underpinning to all research endeavours beyond mere adherence to ethical procedures [71].

Conducting research into sensitive or personal topics such as childbirth experiences and going deeper to reveal stories, emotions, feelings and reflections which they may not have shared with anyone has the potential to be a daunting experience for participants, while the researcher could become immersed in the process and view their stories simply as exciting evidence. The impacts of the research process, participant's reflections and their position in research receive little consideration or acknowledgement which seems unfair as their stories make the evidence for researchers. This issue has been explored by Newton [68] who suggests researchers take an adapting role to respond to the needs, preferences and interests of participants as the research progresses. I grappled with various ethical dilemmas of this kind while conducting my research.

My research followed the procedure of ethics approval and maintained the universal standard of research ethics according to Australia's National Health and Medical Research Council guidelines and approval was sought from the Social and Behavioural Research Ethics Committee of Flinders University of South Australia. In Nepal, I received written permission to conduct the field work from the Family Health Division of the Ministry of Health. In the ethics process, I had to convince the ethics committee to enable a verbal consent process for the research as women in the village were not literate and unable to sign paperwork. I again had to justify to the committee the allowing of a family consent process for the participation of women in the study, as it was culturally appropriate, and women were not allowed to speak with outsiders without the permission of their family. The standard rules, procedures and frameworks associated with ethics processes have limited capacity to take participant's socio-cultural circumstances into account while conducting research [48]. This creates challenges for researchers who are engaged with participants in different social and cultural communities mostly guided by their own social codes, processes and guidelines.

Furthermore, the ethical aspect of the study draws on the concept of deontological morality; the question of whether research treats participants as they ought to be treated or as they have a right to be treated [72]. Schuklenk [73] observed that research lends itself to utilitarian morals within which it should maximise health or satisfaction for the greatest number of people, and in which an action may be justified by its overall results rather than by its effects on individual participants. This perspective, known as consequentialism, is attractive but difficult to maintain practically. Nevertheless, a focus restricted to individual self-determination does not necessarily resonate with our experience of social life, the connectivity between people and the research agenda. I was particularly conscious of my previous connection as an employee in the private sector with health workers and my involvement in maternal health programmes. I tried not to influence participants by bringing these experiences into the research. I made every effort as a researcher to clarify my objectives and role in the research. An incident occurred during field work which illustrates how I maintained my position as a researcher in the village.

> It was my third day in Mugu Village. In the morning, I saw two middle-aged women sitting outside the house. I asked Pasang (the house owner) why these women were sitting there. He said: "they came from another village to see you. Somebody told them that you are a big doctor from another country, and they would like you to assess their problems." I felt surprised, uncomfortable, and sorry for these women. I told them, "I am not a doctor and I can't assess you." I asked them to go to the hospital, which they were not going to do anyway.

Conducting research in complex cross-cultural situations demands a balanced negotiation between researcher and participants around the inherent ethical principles of integrity, respect and justice to accommodate contextual requirements [48]. This involves respecting social and cultural expectations and adapting the research process accordingly. A standard approach to confidentiality, anonymity, informed consent and the researcher-participant relationship does not always work with participants from diverse backgrounds and the researcher needs to make appropriate adjustments according to the situation [4]. For example, in my research it was not possible to maintain the confidentiality of conversations when family members were sharing a common space. As mentioned earlier, in a culture where talking privately with outsiders was not acceptable, I had to accept the presence of other people during interviews.

I made appropriate attempts not to harm research participants, adopting several strategies. Firstly, I gained informed verbal consent with each participant and with their family where necessary. Secondly, I adopted a flexible approach respecting the circumstances by allowing participants to decide where, how and when they would like to have a conversation to share their experiences. Thirdly, participation was made voluntary and interviews were planned as a conversation with no set questions where participants were able to share stories in their own way. Taking a flexible approach enabled participants to take control of what they wanted to tell me, as I used few prompts to let them decide whether to share more or not. Some women stopped the conversation or changed the topic when their husband or mother-in-law or father-in-law appeared. We had to resume our conversation at another time. I acknowledged every encounter and respected decisions that participants made, as they were the ones to know what was right or appropriate to do within their social circumstances.

As Honan et al. [48] point out, maintaining standard ethical codes while respecting localised cultural practices to protect participants without creating social harm during research is complex and challenging for researchers. Managing such complexities to make the right decisions during research was not easy for me but I preserved the aim of privileging people's experiences and respecting their everyday life situations. Indeed, I made every possible effort to maintain the ethics and quality of the research without violating social protocols or creating any harms to the research participants. The flexibility and reflexivity I adopted throughout the research enabled me to gather rich stories in an ethical manner.

Research data: childbirth experiences in everyday life setting

Ongoing debate around the authenticity of data involving personal experiences, everyday life stories and emotions attached to it has been critical to qualitative researchers. The focus in research is on participants' perspectives, actions and emotions, where the researcher becomes an active tool for gathering information and making meaningful interpretations. Social researchers see this as a powerful tool whereas medical researchers disagree. As a feminist researcher, I valued the experiences and stories women shared and the emotions attached to them. When the stories started to become emotional, I grappled with whether I should use my knowledge as an experienced midwife to support them emotionally but stepped away to maintain my status as a researcher. I tried not to assimilate their stories with mine, as the experiences shared by women were unique to the context they were living.

I used face-to-face, in-depth interviews as a method of collecting primary data [74]. This was further supported by field notes which captured thick descriptions of the research setting, the emotions of both participants and the reflections of the researcher. Instead of a structured approach, the interview process applied to a two-way conversation [69], in which the participants were open to share their thoughts, feelings, emotions, stories and experiences of childbirth. Jones and Buggie [75] argue that there is no such thing as assumption-free research, and therefore the researcher should have some broad questions in mind before initiating the interview. Broom [76] suggests having an interview guide to facilitate conversation. I developed an interview guide with broad questions which enabled me to stay in tune with research aims, generate valuable data and maintain the flow of the conversation at the same time.

I used a flexible approach to explore and elaborate on various thoughts, feelings and impressions raised by participants as they identified and talked about different events, moments and incidents in their lives. Initially, I envisaged that this would take the form of a recursive interview model as set out by Minichiello et al. [77], where questioning relies on the process of conversational interaction. Using this technique, I maintained a flexible and reflexive approach, picking up on what was being said at that moment to explore the remark further, or to redirect the participant's focus to the topic of interest. As Denzin and Lincoln [78] point out, reflexive interviews became a concurrently composed discursive method, a site for conversation and a communicative format, enabled to produce knowledge. As a recommended methodological approach in midwifery to demonstrate the trustworthiness of research findings [79], using a reflexive process enabled me to gather detailed insights while making meaning of women's childbirth experiences.

Taylor and Bogdan [80] point out that the relationship between researcher and participant is an essential component of gaining trust while collecting good data. It is understood that the perceptions of both interviewer and participant can influence the nature of discussions during interview [77]. To gain the best possible information from participants, I conducted all interviews engaging in conversation, listening carefully, seeking clarification of concepts as they arose, and asking participants questions about their data when needed. Interviews took place in a location chosen by participants, mostly in their kitchen and working area. I was particularly careful to ensure that the questions were relevant to the language spoken by women. While conversations continued a broad theme, I used to probe to clarify issues further [81]. Oakley [10] suggests using an open style of interviewing in childbirth research, so I kept the conversation open to allow women to talk and share their stories. Our conversations occurred on several occasions over a period to fit in around the women's everyday schedules.

Qualitative interviews provide in-depth and contextualised responses from participants about their views, opinions, feelings, knowledge, emotions and experiences [47]. This type of interview can reveal how certain events impacted participants emotionally which was common in my research as women were sharing stories of losses associated with childbirth. The setting where stories were formed and shared was important to note for a meaningful analysis of the information [49]. I did that by maintaining a reflexive diary which contained not only descriptions of what I had seen and experienced, but also my perceptions and interpretations of these events [82]. This reflexive note taking made me more curious and guided me to obtain a deeper understanding of the socio-cultural situations impacting childbirth experiences of women. I took some photographs, mainly to provide the visual context of the research setting to establish a link with what the women were saying. I utilised the information available in documents and other forms of communication [83], such as policy documents, relevant reports and symbolic scripts to contextualise the experiences participants shared during interviews.

Conducting interviews to elicit the personal childbirth stories of women is not a process of simple conversations. Listening to the experiences of women who have been through a series of perinatal and neonatal losses within complex social circumstances wasn't straightforward as it required patience, the ability to acknowledge the realities and the skills to manage the emotional reactions of both participant and researcher. Although these stories were common for women in the village and they did not seem to have any grief about the continuous losses related to pregnancy or childbirth; it was not easy for me to accept and process them. I felt emotionally exhausted and inundated by the repeated stories of difficult circumstances, neonatal losses and the hardships of everyday life. I was conscious not to make my emotional state visible to participants or demonstrate my reactions to their stories, so stayed calm to composite the experiences shared by women.

Making meaning of lived experiences: analysing childbirth stories

Childbirth stories are personal narratives deeply embedded in the everyday life experiences of women. Collecting the childbirth stories of women living in a complex socio-cultural environment is pivotal to gaining a different perspective by giving importance to the voices of oppressed and marginalised groups [84]. Within a current research approach, a systematic analysis of personal narratives is recommended while making meaning of stories and experiences. Although the childbirth stories of remote mountain women were insightful, appealing and authentic, conducting further analysis of these stories was important to making meaningful interpretations for wider audiences. I reviewed the commonly used methods of qualitative data analysis: thematic analysis [85–87]; grounded theory [88]; and the interpretive phenomenological approach [38, 89]. Having carefully weighed up the benefits and limitations of each one, I decided to use thematic analysis as the appropriate method for this research.

Thematic analysis is compatible with a constructionist approach which is a flexible and useful research tool to provide a rich and detailed account of data within a complex and diverse context [86]. However, Antaki et al. [90] question whether sufficient rigor can be maintained within the inherently flexible approach of thematic analysis. Holloway and Todres [91] confirm that there is no clear agreement among qualitative researchers on the use and effectiveness of the thematic analysis process. Despite these controversies, I felt justified in adopting a thematic analysis approach since it is widely used and fits with the intent of this research [92–96]. There are various thematic analysis processes discussed in the literature; however, I decided to use the strategies provided by Braun and Clarke [86], as they were the most applicable to working through the data I collected for this research.

Thematic analysis is a method for identifying, analysing and reporting themes within the data by exploring various aspects of the research topic and is consistent with a feminist critical approach and values a constructionist view of understanding the meaning of experiences. Emerson et al. [97] argue that the meaning of an event is not transparent but is actively constructed by the participants. Braun and Clarke [86] make it clear that any theoretical framework carries with it several assumptions about the nature of the data in terms of the reality, which can be made transparent through a good thematic analysis. I agree with the primacy of making reality transparent, as it is important to me not to lose the meaning of the stories that women share about their life and childbirth journey.

In a thematic analysis approach, the themes emerge from the data as they are analysed or may have been determined before the analysis began [87]. These two different starting points of analysis are also known as "*inductive*" (data driven) and "*theoretical*" (theory led) thematic analysis [86, 87]. An inductive approach means that themes identified during the analysis process are strongly linked to the data themselves [98] and are not driven by the researcher's theoretical interest in the area [99]. The approach I took in this research was inductive. In doing so, I considered questions of theoretical and epistemological commitment [86], which helped me to enhance the quality of the results.

There are two levels of themes: *"semantic"* and *"latent"* [86]. A semantic approach relies on the explicit and surface meanings of the data, in which the analyst does not look for anything beyond what a participant has said. In contrast, the latent approach examines the underlying ideas, assumptions, conceptualisations and ideologies that are theorised as shaping or informing the semantic content of the data. From a constructionist perspective, meaning and experiences are socially produced and reproduced, rather than inherited within individuals [100]. The latent-level themes provide more material to explore the socio-cultural conditions linking with individual accounts of experiences within a constructivist framework. I focused on latent-level thematic analysis to explore the factors that influence childbirth experiences.

Even though qualitative research is aimed at providing meaningful and valuable results through sophisticated analysis of data, many agree with the fact that there is a lack of appropriate tools to facilitate this process [101–104]. Using the step-by-step process – *familiarising with the data, generating initial codes, searching for the themes, reviewing themes, defining and naming themes, and producing a report* – suggested by Braun and Clarke [86] enabled me to conduct a thorough and systematic analysis of thick narratives to provide meaningful interpretations to the childbirth experiences of women.

Methodological rigor: searching for truth

Qualitative researchers are consistently critiqued for not maintaining the objectivity which would substantiate their claims of methodological rigor. Social researchers believe that reality is multiple and socially constructed and cannot be objectively measured [100, 105, 106]. Thus, rigor in qualitative research involves the careful documentation of social relations, actions and influences [82, 107]. Guba and Lincoln [100] emphasise the importance of trustworthiness in research and suggest five techniques that could be used to assess rigor: *prolonged engagement, persistent observation, triangulation, member checks and auditability.* I used these to assess and maintain methodological rigor in this research.

Prolonged engagement refers to the investment of sufficient time to answer the research questions [100]. I spent three months in each village to gather the data. The time I spent facilitated access to the wide range of actions, interactions and subjective states that were of relevance to developing an in-depth understanding of childbirth experiences of women [41, 108]. I had knowledge of the community, understanding of language and information about maternal and newborn health in the mountains which contributed to the research.

Persistent observation adds the dimension of salience to what might otherwise appear to be little more than a mindless immersion [100]. The field work of this research involved persistent observation in the everyday life setting of participants living in remote mountain villages in Nepal. I lived with a family in the village which provided me with an opportunity to observe everyday events and other happenings. This observation added value to the information collected through the in-depth interviews.

Member checking is an activity in which the researcher takes back the materials to the constructor of the multiple realities under inquiry [100]. In this process, dataset, analytic categories, interpretations and conclusions are tested with the research participants. I offered the opportunity to the participants to check the audio recordings of the interview before transcription and translation into English. I also re-checked the meaning of local terms, asking the person in the field to confirm that the translation maintained the meaning of the actual terms.

Triangulation refers to multiple sources of data, investigators, analysts, multiple ways of interpreting the same set of data or using multiple methods of data collection [100]. Methodological triangulation in this research was done using in-depth interviews, reflective notes of observation and locally available documents as sources of data. Interviews were conducted with women, family members, service providers and local stakeholders to gather their perspectives on pregnancy and childbirth.

Auditability is seen as a means of demonstrating trustworthiness, which refers to the researcher's ability to show a clear decision trail of the progression of events and the researcher's rationale over the life of the study [100]. A successful critique of the auditability of qualitative research is when another researcher clearly follows the decision trail used by the researcher in the study, which might be a description or explanation of a case [108]. In the process of travelling the audit trail, the auditor might focus on field notes that contain personal or methodological information [16]. I maintained reflective field notes which demonstrated the auditability of the research process. As per Sandelowski [106], I provided a clear rationale for the selection of the research topic, recruitment of participants, selection of the research setting, methods for data collection and the analysis process to ensure auditability for research quality.

Hammersley [16] thinks that flexibility in adjusting to changes in circumstances while doing research in the everyday life settings of people provides meaningful understanding of the people's lives and their circumstances. Rice and Ezzy [69] recommend taking a holistic approach to develop a rigorous understanding of the events and data in qualitative research. I maintained rigor from the beginning through developing an appropriate methodology, selecting suitable data collection methods, conducting a reflexive and theoretically informed analysis, and considering ethical aspects of the research.

Stories of women in the Himalayas

Undertaking this challenging journey – transitioning from an academic research centre in Australia to the remote mountain villages of Nepal – was amply rewarded by the opportunity of meeting incredible women who spoke with complete candour both about their astonishing childbirth experiences and their way of life in a remote corner of the world. Most women did not know their age, but instead referenced major past events or calamities – earthquakes, the massacre of the Nepalese royal family or a local pandemic – to estimate how old they were. Those women who did not know their year of birth estimated their ages based on average ages for marriage, first pregnancy and childbirth. For these women, serving the needs of their family, performing household chores and meeting social expectations shaped the boundaries of their lives. The only opportunity for women to expand beyond the confined roles was either to do work assigned to them beyond their daily chores or to get medical help when seriously ill. The childbirth stories women shared with me represent their views about life, their struggles, their resilience and hopes.

Women involved in this research were between the ages of 17 and 43 years, and only one woman was a first-time mother. Among them, only four women had experienced childbirth in a healthcare setting. Out of 20 home births, ten women gave birth in cowsheds and the other ten chose an inside or outside corner of the house. The number of pregnancies each woman had experienced ranged from one to 11, and the age at marriage ranged from 10 to 25 years. Among these pregnancies, there were ten neonatal deaths, seven miscarriages, three stillbirths and one under-five child death with some women experiencing multiple losses. In terms of education, 19 women were illiterate, three had primary-level education, two had completed undergraduate degrees and one had completed a midwifery course. Out of these women, only three had the opportunity of experiencing paid employment.

Women usually walk for days through extraordinarily difficult terrain to reach healthcare workers or a district hospital to access basic health care. Generally, women were living in a shared cottage-type, mud-and-stone house in an extended family structure with their mother-in-law, father-in-law and other family members. In some households, there were 10–15 family members living together in a confined space. Children were mostly sharing a sleeping space with grandparents, while the married couple occupied a space in the corner. Only some women had a semi-private space adjoining the house to share with their spouse. For women living in this way, everything became a shared experience.

Constantly observed, women were cautious about their conversation and activities, aware of the possibility of judgement and censure. In a culture with entrenched inequality along patriarchal lines and strictly defined gender roles enshrined in both religion and custom, women are keenly aware of the penalties for overstepping the boundaries of acceptable female behaviour and are consequently guarded in their behaviours.

Prema

About 29 years old, Prema is a mother of three children. She has been married for 17 years and had her first child at the age of 18. She lost her second baby at nine months. She is currently in the ninth month of her fifth pregnancy. She has had all her births at home with the assistance of her mother-in-law.

Toma

About 26 years old, Toma is a mother of two children. She was married at the age of 20 and had her first baby after a year of marriage. She is currently in the eighth month of her fourth pregnancy. She has had one miscarriage. Toma has had all her previous births at home with the assistance of her mother-in-law.

Lashi

Lashi is 20 years old and is a mother of a newborn baby. She was married at the age of 15 and became pregnant in the same year. She lost her first baby within a month. She gave birth to a second baby two weeks ago. Lashi gave birth at home with the support of her mother-in-law and a neighbouring aunty.

Tolma

About 23 years old, Tolma is a mother of three children. She was married at the age of 13 and two years later, she became pregnant. She has had two miscarriages. Recently, Tolma gave birth to triplets but all of them died within 10 days. She gave birth to all her babies at home with the support of her sister and aunty.

Pema

About 33 years old, Pema was first married at the age of 15 and had a daughter. She left her first husband because of emotional abuse and married another man in the village when she was 20 years old. She has two children with her second husband. She had one miscarriage in the first marriage, and she lost her second baby nine days after its birth in her current relationship. She is due to give birth again next month. Pema gave all births at home with the support of her aunty.

Urgen

About 42 years old, Urgen was married at the age of 14 and is the mother of seven children. She first got pregnant at 17 and is about to give birth to her eighth child. Her daughter-in-law is also pregnant with her first baby and expecting to give birth next month. Urgen gave birth to all her babies at home with the support of her mother.

Dolma

Dolma is 35 years old and is a mother of five children. She was married at the age of 14 and had her first pregnancy at the age of 16. Dolma has experienced one miscarriage, one stillbirth and two neonatal deaths. She lost one three years old child. She is expecting to give birth again in two weeks. For Dolma, all births took place at home with the support of the next-door sister.

Sonam

About 43 years old, Sonam is the mother of three children. She was married at 20 and had her first baby a year after. She has experienced three neonatal losses and one miscarriage. She gave birth last week at the district hospital when serious complications arose. All the other births took place at home with the support of her mother-in-law.

Toli

About 20 years old, Toli is the mother of one child. She was married at the age of 15 and became pregnant a year later. She gave birth to twins, but they died on the ninth and tenth day after their birth. The following year, she gave birth to another baby. Fortunately, that one was alive. She is due to give birth again in two weeks. Toli gave birth to all her babies at home with the help of her mother and aunties.

Jitu

Jitu is about 42 years old and is a mother of seven children ranging in age from five-day-old newborn to 25-year-old youth. She was married at the age of 15 and had her first baby at the age of 16. She lost her 13-year-old son last year due to a wasp sting. Soon she will give birth to her eighth child. She has given birth to all her children at home with the assistance of her mother-in-law and other relatives.

Suntali

Suntali is 24 years old and trained as a midwife. She was married two years ago and has a newborn baby. Her husband is a school teacher working in another district. She gave birth to this baby at the district hospital.

Sunita

Sunita is the only first-time pregnant mother involved in this study. She is 17 years old and is due to give birth in two weeks. Sunita ran away with a school mate two years ago and got married. She has completed primary level schooling. Her husband also dropped out of school after marrying Sunita. She is living with her in-laws and has infrequent prenatal check-ups.

Sanju

Sanju is 18 years old and the mother of two children including a newborn. She also ran away with a school mate when she was in seventh grade and got married when she was only 15. Sanju and her husband did not continue school afterwards. She gave birth both times at the local health post with the assistance from health workers.

Laxmi

Laxmi is about 26 years old and is the mother of three children. She was married at the age of 14 and became pregnant at 16. She is due to give birth to her fourth baby in two weeks. She had all previous births at home with the support of her mother-in-law.

Rama

Rama is about 20 years old and the mother of one child. Rama gave birth to her first baby when she was 17. She had her previous baby at home with the support of her mother-in-law. She is expecting to give birth to her second baby in four weeks at home.

Thuli

About 28 years old, Thuli is a mother of five children. She was married at 13 and gave birth to her first baby at 16. She gave birth to all her babies at home with the support of a local woman. She had experienced one still birth and two neonatal deaths. She had a 25-day-old newborn baby at the time of interview.

Sarita

Sarita is 19 years old and a mother of a newborn baby. She chose to marry a boy in a Maoist camp during the people's war two years ago. She is functionally literate. Sarita gave birth to a preterm baby in the district hospital six days ago with the support of a local midwife.

Manu

About 36 years old, Manu is a mother of seven children. She married at about 14 and had her first baby after two years. Manu has been pregnant 11 times. She has had two miscarriages, and she lost one baby at three months old. Her 11th pregnancy will come to term soon. Manu had all the births at home with support from her mother-in-law.

Hira

About 17 years old, Hira married three years ago. She gave birth to her first child after a year of marriage and lost him before his first birthday. She is currently expecting to give birth to her second baby in four weeks. Her first birth occurred at home with the support of her mother-in-law.

Kiru

About 23 years old, Kiru was married at 14. This is her third pregnancy. Her first baby died the day after its birth. She has one toddler at home. Her previous births occurred at home with the help of her mother-in-law. During this pregnancy she went to the district hospital for a prenatal check-up for the first time but decided to return home to give birth.

Sumi

Sumi is 26 years old and got married at the age of 18. She is a mother of three children. She gave birth to her third baby at the district hospital four days ago. Sumi had two previous babies at home with the support of her mother-in-law. This time she was taken to hospital after a prolonged labour at home.

Rima

Rima is 22 years old and was married at the age of 15. Her first pregnancy ended in miscarriage. Her second pregnancy was delivered by caesarean birth at the city hospital because of complications. She had a planned caesarean two weeks ago and delivered another baby.

Juna

About 40 years old, Juna is a mother of six children. She was married at the age of 10 and gave birth of her first child at the age of 16. She is expecting to give birth to her seventh baby in a week or so. She had all babies at home with the support of her mother-in-law and local women.

Kabita

Kabita is 24 years old and the mother of a three-year-old. She was married at the age of 19 and is working as a primary school teacher at a local primary school. She completed a graduate degree in Education. Kabita is expecting her second child soon. She gave birth to her previous baby at the district hospital and is currently having regular prenatal check-ups.

Rita

Rita is 25 years old and a mother of a five-year-old child. She has completed an undergraduate degree and was working as a school teacher before returning to the village. She married at the age of 19 and gave birth to her first child a year after at a hospital in the city. She is expecting to give birth to her second child in five weeks in the village while her husband is in Qatar for work.

Conclusion

Conducting research in a complex social setting involves managing challenging ethical, moral and methodological complexities. When undertaking research in socially vulnerable and culturally unique communities, researchers can develop fruitful new insights yet simultaneously experience multiple dilemmas. The key issue of maintaining standard ethical processes set by the Western universities when conducting research in culturally and socially diverse populations within the non-Western communities needs close consideration to ensure that research is completed in a safe and respectful way without posing risks to researchers and participants. It is of vital importance that researchers first understand the social circumstances of participants, respecting their status and taking a flexible approach to allow them to adapt to cultural needs, personal preferences, unexpected situations and social-familial expectations.

Researching women's childbirth experiences in complex social and cultural communities requires passion, persistence and patience. Researchers must be able to build trust with women and immerse themselves in their everyday life circumstances. Developing an understanding of differences through building a thorough knowledge of the community where women are and having clear boundaries delineating the position of the researcher could help address insider and outsider dilemmas. Researchers should also adopt an informal, open and natural conversational approach when gathering experiences, allowing women to tell their childbirth stories in their own words.

Reflections drawn from my research experience with women in remote mountains of Nepal provided multiple examples and insights which could serve to enhance understanding of consistently encountered moral, ethical and methodological issues within similarly complex contexts. The socially and culturally adaptable strategies I developed to manage complexities and ethical issues while conducting childbirth research in the most remote and complex social settings in Nepal may well be of benefit to other researchers working within similarly complex circumstances.

References

1   Ember, C.R., *Cross-cultural research methods*. 2009: Rowman & Littlefield, Lanham.
2   Chalmers, B., *Childbirth across cultures: Research and practice*. Birth, 2012. **39**(4): p. 276–280.
3   Davis-Floyd, R.E. and C.F. Sargent, *Childbirth and authoritative knowledge: Cross-cultural perspectives*. 1997: University of California Press, Oakland.
4   Liamputtong, P., *Doing research in a cross-cultural context: Methodological and ethical challenges*, in *Doing cross-cultural research*. 2008: Springer, New York. p. 3–20.
5   Callister, L.C., K. Vehvilainen-Julkunen, and S. Lauri, *Cultural perceptions of childbirth: A cross-cultural comparison of childbearing women*. Journal of Holistic Nursing, 1996. **14**(1): p. 66–78.
6   Pelto, P.J., *Applied ethnography: Guidelines for field research*. 2016: Routledge, London.
7   Baum, F., *The new public health*. 2016: Oxford University Press, Oxford.
8   Wilkinson, S., *Focus groups in health research: Exploring the meanings of health and illness*. Journal of Health Psychology, 1998. **3**(3): p. 329–348.
9   Smith, M.J., *Culture: Reinventing the social sciences*. 2000: Open University Press, Berkshire.

10   Oakley, A., *Interviewing women: A contradiction in terms*. Doing Feminist Research, 1981. **30**(6): p. 1.

11   Oakley, A., *Women confined: Towards a sociology of childbirth*. 1980: Schocken, New York.

12   Bryman, A., *Social research methods*. 2001: Oxford University Press, New York.

13   Brown, S. and J. Lumley, *Changing childbirth: Lessons from an Australian survey of 1336 women*. BJOG: An International Journal of Obstetrics and Gynaecology, 1998. **105**(2): p. 143–155.

14   Larkin, P., C.M. Begley, and D. Devane, *Women's experiences of labour and birth: An evolutionary concept analysis*. Midwifery, 2009. **25**(2): p. e49-e59.

15   Pitchforth, E., et al., *Models of intrapartum care and women's trade-offs in remote and rural Scotland: A mixed-methods study*. BJOG: An International Journal of Obstetrics and Gynaecology, 2008. **115**(5): p. 560–569.

16   Hammersley, M., *What's wrong with ethnography? Methodological explorations*. 1992: Psychology Press, London.

17   Locher, B. and E. Prügl, *Feminism and constructivism: Worlds apart or sharing the middle ground?* International Studies Quarterly, 2001. **45**(1): p. 111–129.

18   Hurley, C., et al., *Comprehensive primary health care in Australia: Findings from a narrative review of the literature*. Australasian Medical Journal, 2010. **1**(2): p. 147–152.

19   Martin, E., *The woman in the body: A cultural analysis of reproduction Milton Keynes*. 1989: Open University Press, Berkshire.

20   Oakley, A., *The captured womb: A history of the medical care of pregnant women*. 1984: Blackwell Publishing, Hoboken.

21   Popay, J. and G. Williams, *Public health research and lay knowledge*. Social Science and Medicine, 1996. **42**(5): p. 759–768.

22   Williams, G. and J. Popay, *Lay knowledge and the privilege of experience*. Challenging Medicine. 1994: Routledge, London. p. 118–139.

23   Van Manen, M., *Phenomenology of practice: Meaning-giving methods in phenomenological research and writing*. 2016: Routledge, London.

24   Savage, J.S., *The lived experience of knowing in childbirth*. The Journal of Perinatal Education, 2006. **15**(3): p. 10.

25   Armstrong, R., et al., *The role and theoretical evolution of knowledge translation and exchange in public health*. Journal of Public Health, 2006. **28**(4): p. 384–389.

26   Popay, J., et al., *A proper place to live: Health inequalities, agency and the normative dimensions of space*. Social Science and Medicine, 2003. **57**(1): p. 55–69.

27   Macintyre, M., *Modernity, gender and mining: Experiences from Papua New Guinea*. Gendering the Field: Towards Sustainable. 2011: ANU Press, Canberra. p. 21–33.

28   Guba, E.G. and Y.S. Lincoln, *Naturalist inquiry*. 1985: Sage Publications, London.

29   Newton, N. and M. Mead, Pregnancy, childbirth, and outcome: A review of patterns of culture and future research needs, in *Childbearing-Its Social and Psychological Aspects*. 1967: Williams and Wilkins, Baltimore.

30   Charon, J.M., *Symbolic interactionism: An introduction, an interpretation, an integration*. 2010: Pearson College Division, London.

31   Burgess, R., *In the field: An introduction to field research*. 1984: Routledge, London.

32   Atkinson, P. and M. Hammersley, *Ethnography: Principles in practice*. 2007: Routledge, New York.

33   Reed-Danahay, D., *Auto/ethnography: Rewriting the self and the social*. 1997: Oxford University Press, Oxford.

34   Schwandt, T.A. and H. Burgon, *Evaluation and the study of lived experience.* The Sage Handbook of Evaluation. 2006: Sage Publications, Thousand Oaks. p. 98–117.

35   Kleinsasser, A.M., *Researchers, reflexivity, and good data: Writing to unlearn.* Theory into Practice, 2000. **39**(3): p. 155–162.

36   Finlay, L. and B. Gough, *Reflexivity: A practical guide for researchers in health and social sciences.* 2008: Wiley and Sons, Hoboken.

37   Finlay, L., *"Outing" the researcher: The provenance, process, and practice of reflexivity.* Qualitative Health Research, 2002. **12**(4): p. 531–545.

38   Heidegger, M., *Being and time (trans: Macquarrie, John and Robinson, Edward).* 1962: Harper and Row, New York.

39   Etherington, K., *Becoming a reflexive researcher: Using ourselves in research.* 2004: Jessica Kingsley Publishers, London.

40   Bell, K., *Doing qualitative fieldwork in Cuba: Social research in politically sensitive locations.* International Journal of Social Research Methodology, 2013. **16**(2): p. 109–124.

41   De Laine, M., *Fieldwork, participation and practice: Ethics and dilemmas in qualitative research.* 2000: Sage Publications, Thousand Oaks.

42   Suwankhong, D. and P. Liamputtong, *Cultural insiders and research fieldwork: Case examples from cross-cultural research with Thai people.* International Journal of Qualitative Methods, 2015. **14**(5): p. 1609406915621404.

43   Caine, K.J., C.M. Davison, and E.J. Stewart, *Preliminary fieldwork: Methodological reflections from northern Canadian research.* Qualitative Research, 2009. **9**(4): p. 489–513.

44   Reeves, C.L., *A difficult negotiation: Fieldwork relations with gatekeepers.* Qualitative Research, 2010. **10**(3): p. 315–331.

45   Shaffir, W. and R.A. Stebbins, *Experiencing fieldwork: An inside view of qualitative research.* Vol. 124. 1990: Sage Publications, Thousand Oaks.

46   Dickson-Swift, V., et al., *Doing sensitive research: What challenges do qualitative researchers face?* Qualitative Research, 2007. **7**(3): p. 327–353.

47   Mikėnė, S., I. Gaižauskaitė, and N. Valavičienė, *Qualitative interviewing: Field-work realities.* 2013: Mykolas Romeris University Press, Vilnious.

48   Honan, E., et al., *Ethical issues in cross-cultural research.* International Journal of Research and Method in Education, 2013. **36**(4): p. 386–399.

49   Mitchell, W. and A. Irvine, *I'm okay, you're okay?: Reflections on the well-being and ethical requirements of researchers and research participants in conducting qualitative fieldwork interviews.* International Journal of Qualitative Methods, 2008. **7**(4): p. 31–44.

50   Chadwick, R., *Embodied methodologies: Challenges, reflections and strategies.* Qualitative Research, 2017. **17**(1): p. 54–74.

51   Acharya, P.P. and D. Rimal, Pregnancy and childbirth in Nepal: Women's role and decision-making power, in *Childbirth across cultures.* 2009: Springer, New York. p. 137–144.

52   Bista, D.B., *The people of Nepal.* 1980: Ratna Pustak Bhandar, Kathmandu.

53   Byrne, A., et al., *Looking beyond supply: A systematic literature review of demand-side barriers to health service utilization in the mountains of Nepal.* Asia Pacific Journal of Public Health, 2013. **25**(6): p. 438–451.

54   Organization, W.H., *Strengthening midwifery within safe motherhood: Report of a collaborative ICM/WHO/UNICEF pre-Congress workshop, Oslo, Norway, 23–26 May 1996.* 1997: World Health Organization.

55 Cameron, M.M., *On the edge of the auspicious: Gender and caste in Nepal*. 1998: University of Illinois Press, Champaign.

56 Dahal, D.R., *Socio-cultural and demographic perspectives of Nepalese women: Problems and issues*. Population Development in Nepal, 1996. **4**: p. 145–155.

57 Panter-Brick, C., *Motherhood and subsistence work: The Tamang of rural Nepal*. Human Ecology, 1989. **17**(2): p. 205–228.

58 Kaphle, S., H. Hancock, and L.A. Newman, *Childbirth traditions and cultural perceptions of safety in Nepal: Critical spaces to ensure the survival of mothers and newborns in remote mountain villages*. Midwifery, 2013. **29**(10): p. 1173–1181.

59 Acharya, S., et al., *Empowering rural women through a community development approach in Nepal*. Community Development Journal, 2005. **42**(1): p. 34–46.

60 Shrestha, S.L., *Gender sensitive planning: What, why, how in Nepal*. 1994: Women Awareness Centre Nepal, Kathmandu.

61 Watkins, J.C., *Spirited women: Gender, religion, and cultural identity in the Nepal Himalaya*. 1996: Columbia University Press, New York.

62 Fisher, J.A., *"Ready-to-recruit" or "ready-to-consent" populations? Informed consent and the limits of subject autonomy*. Qualitative Inquiry, 2007. **13**(6): p. 875–894.

63 Munford, R. and J. Sanders, *Recruiting diverse groups of young people to research: Agency and empowerment in the consent process*. Qualitative Social Work, 2004. **3**(4): p. 469–482.

64 Tyldum, G., *Ethics or access? Balancing informed consent against the application of institutional, economic or emotional pressures in recruiting respondents for research*. International Journal of Social Research Methodology, 2012. **15**(3): p. 199–210.

65 Kapoulas, A. and M. Mitic, *Understanding challenges of qualitative research: Rhetorical issues and reality traps*. Qualitative Market Research: An International Journal, 2012. **15**(4): p. 354–368.

66 Karnieli-Miller, O., R. Strier, and L. Pessach, *Power relations in qualitative research*. Qualitative Health Research, 2009. **19**(2): p. 279–289.

67 Morse, J.M., *Qualitative nursing research: A contemporary dialogue*. 1990: Sage Publications, Thousand Oaks.

68 Newton, V.L. *'It's good to be able to talk': An exploration of the complexities of participant and researcher relationships when conducting sensitive research. in Women's Studies International Forum*. 2017. Elsevier, Amsterdam.

69 Rice, P.L. and D. Ezzy, *Qualitative research methods: A health focus*. 1999: Oxford University Press, Sydney.

70 Davis, D.L. and K. Walker, *Re-discovering the material body in midwifery through an exploration of theories of embodiment*. Midwifery, 2010. **26**(4): p. 457–462.

71 Hansen, E., *Successful qualitative health research*. 2006: Allen and Unwin, Sydney.

72 Osrin, D., et al., *Ethical challenges in cluster randomized controlled trials: Experiences from public health interventions in Africa and Asia*. Bulletin of the World Health Organization, 2009. **87**: p. 772–779.

73 Schüklenk, U., *Protecting the vulnerable: Testing times for clinical research ethics*. Social Science and Medicine, 2000. **51**(6): p. 969–977.

74 Sarantakos, S., *Social research*. 2012: Macmillan International Higher Education, London.

75 Jones, A. and C. Bugge, *Improving understanding and rigour through triangulation: An exemplar based on patient participation in interaction*. Journal of Advanced Nursing, 2006. **55**(5): p. 612–621.

76   Broom, A., *Using qualitative interviews in CAM research: A guide to study design, data collection and data analysis*. Complementary Therapies in Medicine, 2005. **13**(1): p. 65–73.

77   Minichiello, V., R. Aroni, and T.N. Hays, *In-depth interviewing: Principles, techniques, analysis*. 2008: Pearson Education, Sydney.

78   Denzin, N.K. and Y.S. Lincoln, *The Sage handbook of qualitative research*. 2011: Sage Publications, Thousand Oaks.

79   Kingdon, C., *Reflexivity: Not just a qualitative methodological research tool*. British Journal of Midwifery, 2005. **13**(10): p. 622–627.

80   Taylor, S.J. and R. Bogdan, *Introduction to qualitative research methods: The search for meanings*. 1984: Wiley Inter-Science, Hoboken.

81   Berg, B.L., *Qualitative research methods for the social science*. 2007: California State University, Long Beach.

82   Liamputtong, P., *Qualitative data analysis: Conceptual and practical considerations*. Health Promotion Journal of Australia, 2009. **20**(2): p. 133–139.

83   Bryman, A., *Social research methods*. 2016: Oxford University Press, Oxford.

84   Callister, L.C., *Making meaning: Women's birth narratives*. Journal of Obstetric, Gynaecologic and Neonatal Nursing, 2004. **33**(4): p. 508–518.

85   Attride-Stirling, J., *Thematic networks: An analytic tool for qualitative research*. Qualitative Research, 2001. **1**(3): p. 385–405.

86   Braun, V. and V. Clarke, *Using thematic analysis in psychology*. Qualitative Research in Psychology, 2006. **3**(2): p. 77–101.

87   Hayes, N., *Doing psychological research*. 2000: Buckingham, Open University Press, Berkshire.

88   Glaser, B.G. and A.L. Strauss, *Discovery of grounded theory: Strategies for qualitative research*. 2017: Routledge, London.

89   Gadamer, H.-G., *1999. Truth and Method*. 1960: Continuum International Publishing Group, New York.

90   Antaki, C., et al., *Discourse analysis means doing analysis: A critique of six analytic shortcomings*. Discourse Analysis Online, 2003.

91   Holloway, I. and L. Todres, *The status of method: Flexibility, consistency and coherence*. Qualitative Research, 2003. **3**(3): p. 345–357.

92   Banning, M., et al., *The impact of culture and sociological and psychological issues on Muslim patients with breast cancer in Pakistan*. Cancer Nursing, 2009. **32**(4): p. 317–324.

93   Bayes, S., J. Fenwick, and Y. Hauck, *A qualitative analysis of women's short accounts of labour and birth in a Western Australian public tertiary hospital*. Journal of Midwifery and Women's Health, 2008. **53**(1): p. 53–61.

94   Berman, R.C. and L. Wilson, *Pathologizing or Validating: Intake Workers' Discursive Constructions of Mothers*. Qualitative Health Research, 2009. **19**(4): p. 444–453.

95   Clarke, S.-A., L. Sheppard, and C. Eiser, *Mothers' explanations of communicating past health and future risks to survivors of childhood cancer*. Clinical Child Psychology and Psychiatry, 2008. **13**(1): p. 157–170.

96   Souza, J.P., et al., *An emerging "maternal near-miss syndrome": Narratives of women who almost died during pregnancy and childbirth*. Birth, 2009. **36**(2): p. 149–158.

97   Emerson, R.M., R.I. Fretz, and L.L. Shaw, *Writing ethnographic fieldnotes*. 2011: University of Chicago Press, Chicago.

98   Patton, M.Q., *Qualitative evaluation and research methods*. 1990: Sage Publications, Thousand Oaks.

99 Hayes, N., *Doing psychological research*. 2000: Open University Press, Buckingham.

100 Lincoln, Y.S. and E.G. Guba, *Naturalistic inquiry (vol. 75)*. 1985: Sage Publications, Thousand Oaks.

101 Denzin, N.K. and Y.S. Lincoln, *Collecting and interpreting qualitative materials*. 2008: Sage Publications, Thousand Oaks.

102 Huberman, A.M. and M.B. Miles, *Data management and analysis methods*. 1994: Sage Publications, Thousand Oaks.

103 Lee, R.M. and N. Fielding, *Qualitative data analysis: Representations of a technology: A comment on Coffey, Holbrook and Atkinson*. Sociological Research Online, 1996. 1(4): p. 15–20.

104 Silverman, D., *Doing qualitative research: A practical handbook*. 2013: Sage Publications, Thousand Oaks.

105 Morse, J.M., *"Going beyond your data," and other dilemmas of interpretation*. 2009: Sage Publications, Thousand Oaks.

106 Sandelowski, M., *The call to experts in qualitative research*. Research in Nursing and Health, 1998. 21(5): p. 467–471.

107 Ratner, C., *Solidifying qualitative methodology*. Journal of Social Distress and the Homeless, 1996. 5(3): p. 319–326.

108 De Laine, M., *Ethnography: Theory and applications in health research*. 1997: MacLennan and Petty, Sydney.

4 Tradition, culture and spirituality
God inside

Introduction

> I have always given birth in the Goth [Cow Shed]. Where should I give birth other than the Goth? In your place [referring to where I come from], you may give birth at home or hospital, but here we don't do that. We have Deuta [God] inside the house. We shouldn't be doing wrong things or polluting the house. If we do so, our baby might die or something wrong might happen to the family or to our animals. So, we prefer the Goth to give birth and to keep the house clean. I stayed in the Goth for a month after the birth. I am doing the right thing. You know, the next door Kanchi [referring to another woman] went inside the house on her fourth day of Chau [menstruation] and her baby fell sick. I might've touched something to make God angry, you know I lost two babies in the Goth [takes a long breath]. This is not good if God gets angry . . . we may die, and it won't help us. We should never make God angry. Thuli

Mary Douglas provides important insight into the universal phenomenon of purity and pollution beliefs, connecting them ultimately to the ethnic and cultural ideas of social order and the danger inherent in its reproduction [1]. Her model remains useful in a variety of cultural contexts in Nepal, where beliefs about pollution during childbirth tend to be embedded in childbirth practices. She proposes that pollution beliefs operate at two levels: instrumental and expressive. At the instrumental level, people in mountain villages in Nepal claim that certain illnesses and deaths may be caused by pollution transgressions. To prevent these unwanted outcomes, women must take care not to violate pollution-based codes of conduct during and after childbirth. At the expressive level, pollution beliefs symbolise the social order of people. The impurity of women's childbirth is controlled through the moral order of deity (Dharma) and the honour of patriline.

The custom that women remain isolated in cowsheds during delivery and for up to 30 days after childbirth is common in most of the mountain villages. Embedded traditions, culture and spiritual beliefs inform childbirth as a socio-cultural event, as illustrated by women's experiences of giving birth. The main reason that women refer to, and has emerged from research, is the supernatural powers affecting childbirth. Women called it God's power or God's will. The word "Deuta" is a collective term that villagers use to refer to a range of Gods and Goddesses. The belief that God's will is the primary cause that determines health and illness is a commonly shared view in both Buddhist and Hindu communities in the mountains. For all women, their families and the communities, the role of "Deuta" is significant to determine childbirth outcomes.

Never been outside: empowering self and maintaining safety

"Where did you give birth to your previous babies, Toma Sister?" I asked.

"I always give birth in the Goth. I have never been outside the Goth to give birth. Did you see the Goth next to our house when you visited yesterday? That is where I gave birth," Toma responded.

Demonstrating the concept of empowerment [2], women's capacity to make choices about the way they give birth enables them to take control of their childbirth. This not only allows women to maintain their traditions but also ensures their cultural safety. One example of this is the practice of giving birth in cowsheds, known locally as Goth. A Goth is the preferred birthing place of many women. One corner of the Goth is used to accommodate women during menstruation,

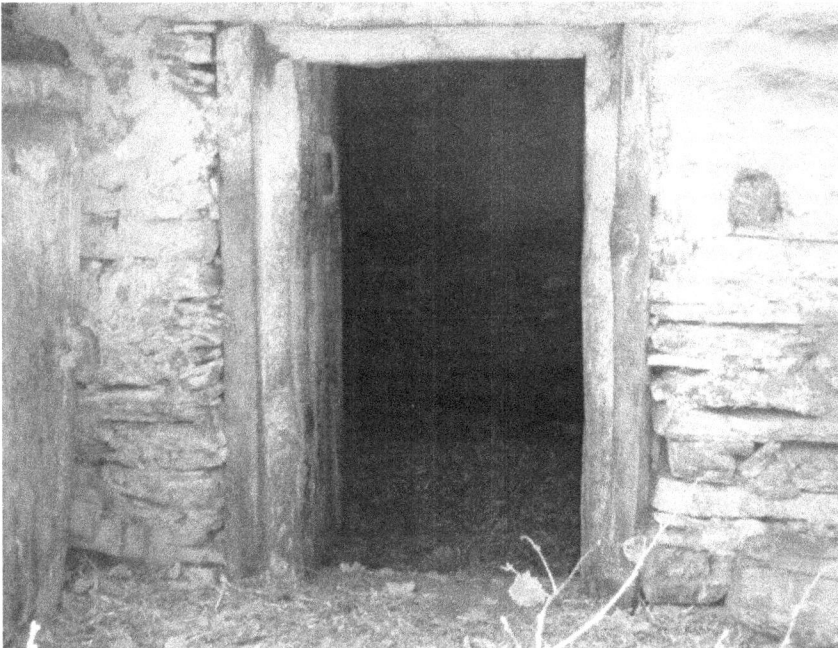

Figure 4.1 The Goth – where women give birth and spend polluted days

Source: Picture taken by the author

childbirth and the postnatal period. The Goth is normally part of the ground floor of a two-storey house or an adjoining hut built from mud and stone. It is a dark space with a low ceiling, a very narrow door and no window. The entrance is directly from outside, and the building does not connect with the rest of the house. It does not have a lockable door.

Giving birth in the Goth is dictated by the perceived polluting nature of the childbirth. The seclusion of women during birth is an attempt to protect the woman and others around her from danger by safeguarding them from pollution. While giving birth in seclusion in the Goth, women are not allowed to have any contact with other family members. Only her close female kin or TBAs are permitted to support the birthing process. In traditional Nepalese societies, the first 30 days after the birth are considered the polluting period when women are kept in isolation.

Remote mountain women shared their reasons for giving birth in the Goth and explained their preference to maintain this tradition. Continuing the practice was significant to them because they believe that it ensures no one dies or falls sick in the family due to birth pollution. As Thuli indicated above, according to tradition and spiritual beliefs, the practice of giving birth in the Goth is the correct standard to follow to minimise the chances of experiencing negative birth outcomes.

Toma shared a similar view.

> Both times, I gave birth in Goth. Baby came without a trouble. I didn't have any problems. Giving birth wasn't hard at all. We all know that it is normal to have some pain and discomfort while giving birth. Other women in the villages also give birth in Goth. We think this is the right thing to do. For us, giving birth is an easy and simple task. It is our tradition to stay in Goth and we believe that Goth is the only safe place to give birth in our village. Toma

The perception of childbirth as a normal, easy and simple task contributed to the cultural norms governing the place of birth for women. Toma talked about the universality of birthing in the Goth, and she indicated her respect for both cultural practice and traditional knowledge through maintaining cultural expectations. Women and the villagers regarded childbirth in the Goth as the best practice to minimise the risks to mother and baby.

Manu expressed her feeling of lacking safety when she had to move away from the Goth.

> When I went to the hospital last time, they [doctors] told me that the baby is okay. I didn't feel like staying in the hospital anymore. It wasn't the place for me. I had no desire to give birth there. The next morning: I left the hospital, went to my sister's house, and gave birth at her Goth. Nothing wrong happened – everything went well – the baby was fine. Later I thought, I shouldn't have gone to the hospital leaving other children behind. Up until now, I gave all births in the Goth. This time, I am determined not to go to the hospital. I am happy being in the Goth and following our valued tradition. Manu

Manu linked the preference for giving birth in the Goth to her cultural connections to the practice which influenced her perception of safety. She did not have the same feeling of safety in the hospital and eventually became determined to return to a familiar environment to give birth. For Manu, childbirth in the Goth was the best option and her preferred choice.

For remote mountain women, childbirth is a collective experience. In the conversations, women referred to the involvement of others and for Manu it was her sister who allowed her to give birth in her Goth. In the collective understanding, childbirth in the Goth is associated with positive experiences of exercising agency by continuing traditional practices. These notions of collectivism, agency and control are apparent when Juna explains how births usually occur in the Goth and the traditions attached to the practice.

> We always give birth at Goth. First, we clean the Goth and then we put straw on the floor. We give birth on this straw. We burn the straw that has blood on it. We put clean straws in the Goth to sleep on it, and we stay there with the baby for 20–30 days after giving birth. We make a fire and keep it going so the baby stays warm. This is our usual practice when giving birth. I always stayed in Goth for 30 days after the childbirth. Some women come out after 20 days. We can touch water on 30th day and are permitted to go inside the house. We go through a special purification process by Bahun [Priest] on the 30th day. I felt so happy coming out from Goth without any problems. There was no sickness in the family – not to the baby or the other members. I never did the wrong thing, so God is happy to help me all the time. Juna

Juna's sense of doing the correct thing by meeting cultural expectations is an example of how safety is perceived by women during childbirth. Validating the belief system and traditional knowledge by giving birth inside the Goth and following the pollution practices by remaining confined after the birth has intergenerational significance in childbirth culture in the mountains. The older generation mothers-in-law were happy about the continuation of tradition.

Juneli, a mother-in-law, expressed her satisfaction with younger women continuing childbirth traditions.

> All the time, I gave birth while I was working in the field. My middle one was born while I was cropping potatoes. I came home with the baby wrapped in a shawl and went straight to the Goth. I can't compare my stories these days. We stayed in Goth for a month after the birth of the baby. I am happy that my oldest daughter-in-law [Jethi Buhari] lives with me and is still giving birth in the same Goth. The traditions are the same in the village and we like to maintain it. Juneli

Another mother-in-law, Chameli highlighted why the childbirth tradition in Goth is important.

> We always gave birth in Goth. We shouldn't give birth inside the house. We don't go inside the house for five days during menstruation [Chau] either. We are afraid bad results could happen if we go inside the house or accidently touch the Deuta [God]. So, we can't let our daughters-in-law give birth inside the house. That is not going to happen in our time in this village. We must take them to the Goth. We have been following the same tradition, as our mothers and mothers-in-law did. We want our daughters-in-law to do the same. Following the traditions is better than taking risks of experiencing multiple problems afterwards. Chameli

"Bad results" refer to the possibility of causing death and sickness through not following the tradition. These women expressed a strong determination to continue traditions and respect pollution beliefs in order to minimise the risks of childbirth pollution associated deaths or sickness. Their experiences of childbirth inside the Goth without "bad results" facilitated the continuity of the practice from one generation to another. From their perspective, coming out of the Goth to give birth would threaten their survival during and after the childbirth. Believing in the likelihood of bad things happening because of breaking the cultural norms, women are highly motivated to continue the tradition of childbirth in the Goth.

Women remain confined after childbirth and are not allowed to touch anything during the pollution period. This includes people, animals, plants and places. There is a belief that the polluted touch causes deaths or sickness or other undesirable outcomes. Women are not allowed to go outside the Goth during this period.

A 26-year-old male traditional faith healer mentioned why traditions are hard to change.

> Giving birth in the Goth is our tradition. We consider that women become impure [Chau] during childbirth. They can't touch any people or go inside the house during and after the childbirth. This deeply rooted traditional beliefs of society are making things difficult for women. I took my wife on the third day after birth inside the house during her second time. However, other people from the village made comments and they did not like what I did. They complained about it and blamed me for taking this action and causing harms to others by violating tradition. Because of that social blame, I had to send her back to the Goth. I didn't have courage to break the traditional practice and bring her inside the house afterwards. Though I wanted her to come home and stay comfortable, it wasn't acceptable to the society. Traditional faith healer

There is a difference between how women and the traditional faith healer view the childbirth traditions. The faith healer's attempt to act contrary to tradition is opposed to the preference of the women who feel safer remaining in the Goth. This provides a critical insight in understanding cultural norms and shows how traditional social values can limit individual attempts to initiate change in a collectivist community.

A male local health worker confirmed that the tradition of birth in the Goth has a significant place in the society.

> Honestly speaking, the reasons for giving birth in Goth are attached to the religious belief and with Gods and Goddesses. One reason is related to untouchability in which family members shouldn't touch childbearing birthing, and postnatal women. Another reason is because many people have only a common space in their home, which they can't make impure by allowing women when they are polluted. As a result, they must go to the Goth to give birth. In the Goth, there is no ventilation and light, but they can light a fire to stay warm. Having their own space and being able to light a fire is a good thing for both mother and baby. The older generation people understand this way. The practice of giving birth in Goth is related to the lack of health education also. Our people [indicating villagers] don't know about science and they continue to believe in old traditions. I can say that modern people [youth] are also not ready to change the tradition that has been practiced for many generations. Local health worker

The health worker shared a different view of the childbirth traditions associating them with a lack of education. He admitted the reality of the continuation of traditional practices that impose restrictions on women based on religion and traditional beliefs. However, he blamed the older generation for keeping the practice strong and ensuring its continuity in the younger generation. There is a clear distinction between the perspective of the women and the local health worker around childbirth traditions.

It is not surprising that health workers considered childbirth in the Goth as an unsafe practice. However, the critique made by health workers of the use of Goth as the birthing place does not seem logical or practical to those women who have no other place to choose for childbirth.

Urgen described the tensions of balancing social, cultural and medical expectations.

> We don't have a health centre or a hospital nearby. We don't have other rooms in the house where we can give birth and stay afterwards. We don't have any options, so we go to the Goth. Though it is not safe as they [health workers] said, we will be giving birth in the Goth for years to come. They [health workers] told us to have regular check-ups, nutritious food and take better care. Do they not realise that we don't have a place to go for check-ups, we don't have enough food to eat and we don't have time to take a rest? They can't just come and tell us what to do. Urgen

As discussed previously, the Government of Nepal has adopted a medical discourse in their intervention strategies. This discourse views childbirth as a high-risk event and considers medical care for women experiencing complications as the only option for mitigating the risk [3]. Urgen shared her frustration that health workers used the power of medical discourse to insist women take actions which were not feasible for them. This indicated a lack of understanding by the health workers of the social context of mountain women's lives and an inability to consider the implications of this context on their choices. There is a failure by medical practitioners to design and deliver relevant and helpful information.

I spoke with the medical doctor working in the district hospital to get his perspective on the tradition of giving birth in the Goth. The doctor cited culture and tradition as a big problem in the village which is putting both mother and the babies at risk of dying.

> Giving birth in Goth is the reality in the district, I can't deny that. This is the tradition here. It has been practiced for many years. We can't change culture and tradition in a single day or in a single year. However, the trend of giving birth in health institutions is improving in recent years but it isn't to the same level where we wanted to be. So, we are running various programs and we are raising awareness of people about the danger of having births in the Goth and about the risks of infections, neonatal tetanus and all these things. We are telling them to do the right thing by coming to the hospital for check-ups and to give births. Medical doctor

The doctor has adopted the medical risk approach, but his view does not consider the socio-cultural significance of childbirth and the associated notion of safety expressed by the women. For women, remaining in the village, continuing the tradition of giving birth in the Goth and following the 30 days pollution practice was "doing the right thing." The medical doctor held a perspective opposed to the preferences and choices of women in their attempts to prevent risks which he believes can only be mitigated if women go to hospital. Different concepts of safety proposed by the medical and cultural domains are incompatible and create a serious dilemma for women to negotiate.

On the one side, women are not willing to leave the Goth because they believe that remaining there keeps them safe, and on the other side, the doctor wants to bring them to the hospital to give birth because this is how he believes their safety will be best ensured. The medical paradigm needs to acknowledge the importance of cultural norms pertaining to childbirth because ignoring it undermines the sense of safety and agency that women need to retain during childbirth. There is a need for collaborative practice bringing the aspects of both medical and socio-cultural models to lower the risk and to promote the sense of safety while giving birth.

Disregard of the social context and sense of safety during childbirth by the health workers and the medical discourse was further confirmed by a local FCHV who outlined the difficulties that women would experience if they go to hospital to give birth, as maintaining the culture and tradition is still their priority.

> While we help women giving birth in the Goth, they do not allow us to touch them [support person] after the baby is born. We consider the mother impure. We follow the tradition, belief and practices of not touching during the birth

pollution period, normally 30 days. Asking them to go to hospital to give birth isn't good in this context. If women go to the health post or hospital to give birth, they need to carry their stuff and the baby on the way back home, as other people are not allowed to touch. They don't like doing that, it's a big load when they are already weak and exhausted to walk home with. Instead, they prefer staying home and going inside the Goth to give birth and to spend their 30 days. I also gave all my births at Goth. I did the same as other women do in the village to maintain the tradition. Female community health volunteer

The FCHV valued tradition. Even though she was a trained health worker and understood the risks and complications associated with traditional childbirth practices, she did not practice childbirth differently to other women in the village. Maintaining purity by following the birth pollution practice remained the focus for her. The FCHV also highlighted some of the physical impracticalities of going to hospital to give birth which contribute to local women's lack of motivation.

An interplay between various socio-cultural factors in shaping childbirth practice was evident in the women's experiences. Both Hindu and Buddhist women shared the pollution belief and followed the tradition. The local Indigenous leader spoke about the collective practice.

In Lama culture, we don't have any written codes or religious concept of birth pollution that restricts women to give birth inside the house. However, Lama families also follow the same pollution practice that others do, which means they don't give birth inside the house. Lama women also go to the Goth. The Hindu concept of birth pollution has been mixed with Lama culture in the village which is restricting women going inside the house to give birth and for certain days after the childbirth. Community is following the culture more than the religion. People are moving houses, but the childbirth pollution practice is not changing. This pollution belief has influenced the practice of everyone in the same way. Local Indigenous leader

This is an example of a transfer of ideas between different cultures and groups that inform a unified perspective on childbirth practice in the mountains. The universal notions governing childbirth in the Goth among both Hindu and Lama women indicates the possibility that the medical and cultural views be brought together to ensure positive experiences for women. Shared values and mutual understanding among the members of the group often govern which decisions an individual makes. That individual decisions are based on the collective values so that women stay within the group's cultural norms [4] is common when it comes to culture and tradition governing to childbirth in these villages.

A school teacher from the local primary school emphasised how this collective social construct is embedded in the childbirth tradition in these villages.

There have been no changes in the tradition since I came here [23 years ago] because they are giving more value to their cultural practices. In the village where I have been working for several years now, women can touch the water only on the sixth day of their menstruation and on 30th day after the child-birth. As you have already been to the other villages, you would be aware of their tradition of giving birth in Goth and living in Goth after menstrua-tion and childbirth. This is an intergenerational tradition and everyone in the village follows it with respect. This tradition exists even in the family of educated members. It is commonly accepted and highly respected practice in these villages. School teacher

The school teacher made it clear that people in these villages give more value to their tradition than the new information they receive from other sources. The criticism by the health worker of the local people's ignorance in valuing tradition needs further discussion given in one example cited here, an educated person also did not prefer the traditional childbirth practice. This collective adherence to culture and tradition with the intention of enhancing the safety of mothers, babies and families is an important aspect of women's childbirth experiences in these remote mountain villages.

Furthermore, the interaction of culture, tradition and spiritual practice deter-mined the sense of safety these women experienced during childbirth. It was clear that their cultural and spiritual beliefs shaped their understanding of childbirth. For them, the tradition of birth in the Goth was significant and continuing that practice made childbirth an empowering experience for them. The persistence of pollution beliefs restricts willingness to accept the medical model; women make their own decisions about what to do to make birth comfortable, how the birth could be safe and who to call for help if assistance was required. This capacity to make decisions allowed them to have collective ownership and agency during childbirth experiences.

The socio-cultural conditions in which women live influence their birthing experiences. These circumstances that shape the women's lives also affect child-birth outcomes. The analysis of cultural dimensions of childbirth has been over-shadowed universally in the current era by the powerful domain of medicalised childbirth [5]. The limitations of the medical approach in ensuring community ownership of the childbirth experiences of women are evident in these stories. As Labonte [6] argues, the medical model is concerned with high-risk individu-als, women felt a lack of consideration of their socio-cultural circumstances in the hospital. The experiences women shared highlighted the value they place on tradition and the importance of following their cultural norms during childbirth.

These women in the remote mountains were committed to their confinement in the Goth when giving birth and during the 30 days pollution period. From the spiritual point of view, this practice was important for keeping mothers and babies safe from illness or unexpected deaths. Under these circumstances, differences in understanding of risk and safety contained in cultural and medical practices created a critical disjunction between the ways the two practices seek to ensure maternal and newborn survival. Care providers should make efforts to develop mutual understanding while providing care taking both cultural and medical measures to address the complex needs of women around childbirth practices.

Oakley [7] highlights the importance of culture and tradition in ensuring well-being in childbirth, women expressed the feeling of being safe while giving birth inside the Goth. Although they sometimes experienced the loss of newborn babies while giving birth in the Goth, they felt that following the practice of childbirth pollution was more important than the deaths of the newborn. Nepalese women in rural areas experiencing childbirth in the Goth often felt dehumanised [8]. However, the women accepted this tradition and felt that giving birth in the Goth enhanced their perception of safety and collective ownership of the childbirth.

Better than polluting: negotiated practice and respect for tradition

Childbirth in many societies is seen as a polluting event [9]. Consistent with Callister et al. [10], remote mountain women view childbirth as a significant spiritual event. Women associated the practice of not giving birth inside the house and remaining outside during the childbirth pollution to their spiritual beliefs. Rice et al. [11] describe Hmong women's in South East Asia the feeling of being spiritually unsafe while experiencing childbirth in a hospital setting. A few women in this study also felt culturally threatened while they were in hospital and two women returned home to give birth traditionally.

While respecting tradition, women were able to negotiate a birthplace outside the Goth. Their ability to negotiate shows that culture and tradition are not absolute and static practices wherein individuals had no agency, but that there is the possibility for change. Nevertheless, this negotiation of the birthplace occurred without changing the determination to follow accepted pollution practice during the birth and postnatal days. Women shared how the tradition of birth inside the Goth was negotiated in practice.

The outside corner that women mentioned was a space adjoining the common family area on the first floor of the house. This was another place that some women used to give birth and spend their polluted days. Participants maintained a similar level of respect for their pollution beliefs and still did not go inside the house during and after the birth. This birthplace allowed the women to remain confident they were keeping God's place (inside the house) clean to ensure safety.

Toma maintained tradition by remaining in the corner of the house to protect from birth pollution.

> We have Deuta [God] inside the house. We are afraid of the pollution. We shouldn't be polluting God's place. If we do so, something bad will happen either for the baby or for the mother or for the other members of the family. We aren't allowed to go upstairs or inside the house to give birth. I don't like polluting the God's place. So, I gave all the births in the corner outside. Toma

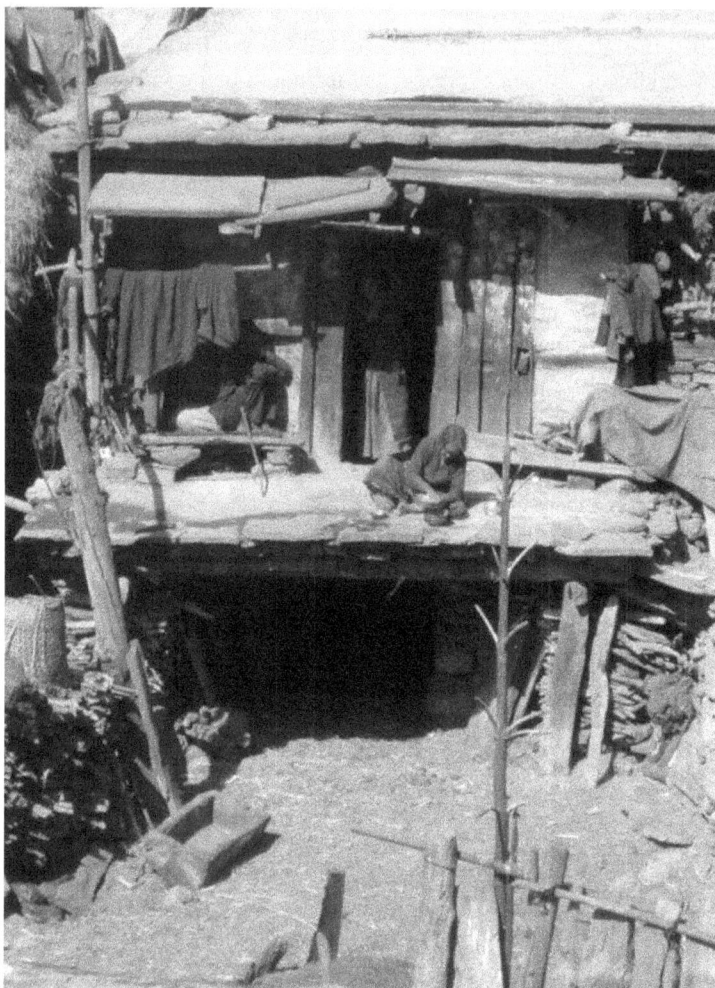

Figure 4.2 The outside corner – where women give birth and spend polluted days
Source: Picture taken by the author

While some women gave birth in the outside corner, some others could give birth in the inside corner of the house. A typical mountain home is usually two storeys, where the first floor is shared by the family for all purposes and the ground floor is used to house animals. The inside corner of the house that women referred to is the space next to the animal shed which they used to give birth and spend the pollution days.

The conversation with Jitu explored the inside corner of the house as a preferred place to give birth.

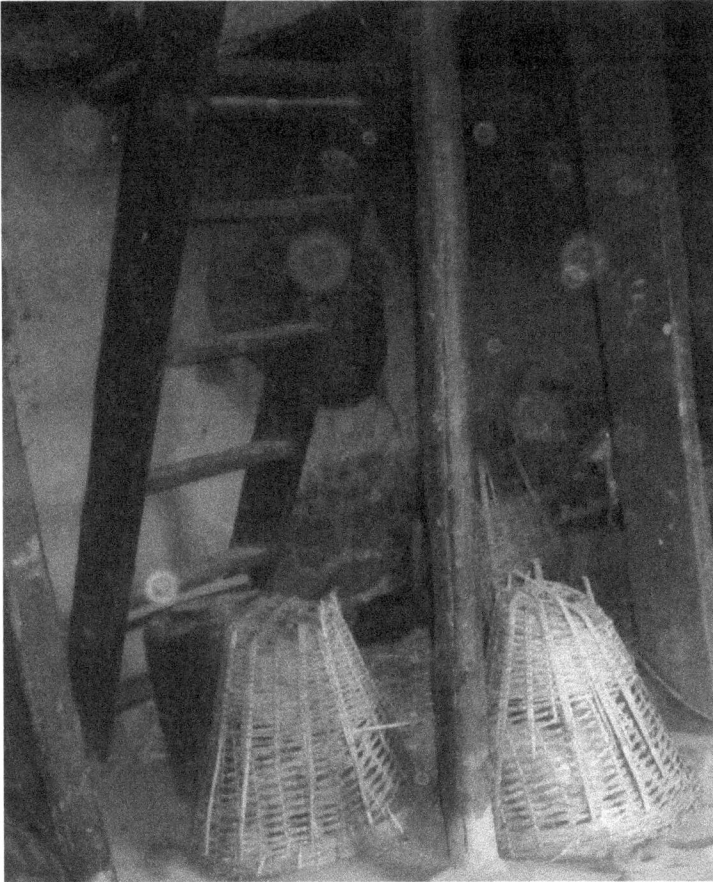

Figure 4.3 The inside corner – where women give birth and spend polluted days
Source: Picture taken by the author

Where did you give birth to Jitu Didi?
Where? Of course, at home. Where would it be if not home? She laughed and
    questioned back.
Where at home did you give birth?
I never went to Goth to give birth. I gave birth downstairs in the corner where the
    fire oven is. I like to be there as I can put on the fire to keep the baby warm and
    I am still away from God's place, she responded.
Was it easy to give birth there?
I never had problems. Baby just comes when it is time. Jitu smiled.

Keeping God happy, seeing childbirth as an easy process and ensuring the comfort
of the baby were the accomplishments that Jitu was proud of in giving birth. This

consciousness of spirituality and cultural beliefs underlies the women's ability to articulate the reasons for their preferences and continuity of tradition.

Similar negotiation about the birthplace occurred for Laxmi. Her mother-in-law, Hira, allowed her daughters-in-law to remain in a room attached to the house. Hira recalled her birthing experiences and compared it with the current practice.

> During our time, we gave all births in the Goth. They [family and community] didn't allow us to go inside the house to give birth. In the village, other women are still giving birth in Goth. In my house, as my sons are educated, they didn't let us give birth in the Goth, so I took my daughter in law to the

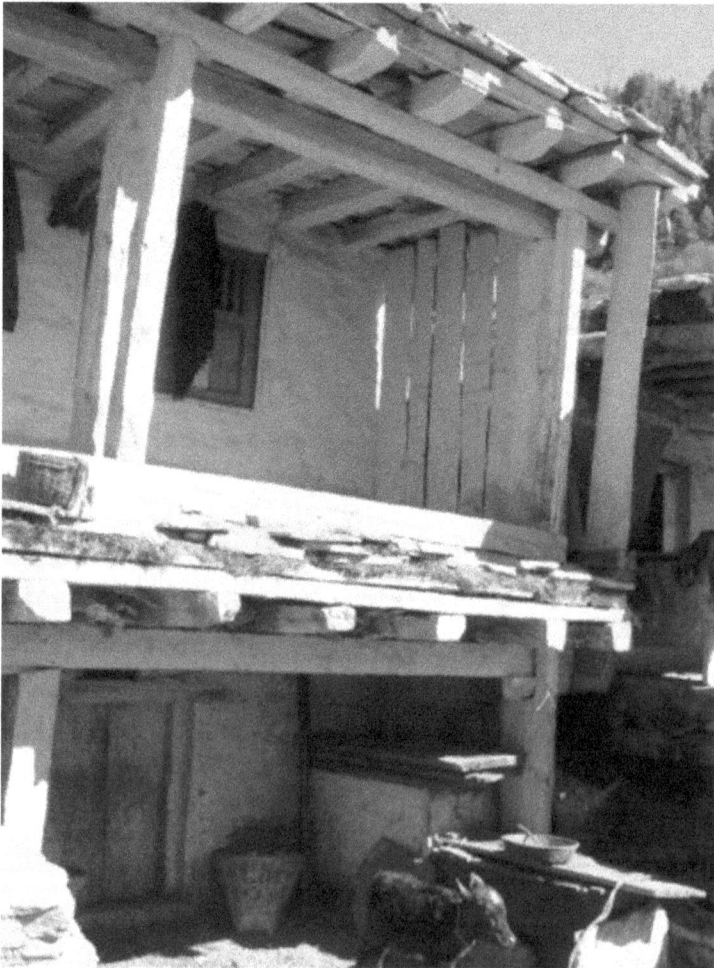

Figure 4.4 A separate room – where women give birth and spend postnatal days

Source: Picture taken by the author

room downstairs. It has made their birth better and I was happy that we were still able to maintain tradition. Hira

Hira's reflections show that the culture and tradition are changing over time which enabled her to now avoid births in the Goth. However, the room she referred to is still connected to the cowshed but with a door to separate it from the room. Sumi, the daughter-in-law affirmed the practice of being confined to a separate room to give birth and to spend the 30 polluted days.

We don't have that system of giving birth in the Goth. This tradition has changed. I had the first two births in the same room outside the house. We don't give birth inside [referring to common family areas]. It isn't good to go inside during Chau [polluted time]. I always stayed outside in this room [a room made of mud and stone without windows on the ground floor of the house usually used for keeping wood] to give birth and for a month after the birth. Even my mother-in-law stays there during her Chau [menstruation] for four days. Sumi

Sumi was able to be out of the Goth during childbirth but still maintained a sense of good practice and did not violate cultural expectations. The dialogue between traditional and medical knowledge to achieve safe childbirth experiences was possible for Suntali, who is a trained midwife.

I gave birth in the hospital. According to our tradition, they didn't allow me to go inside the house without performing rituals to become pure. After the birth, I came home and stayed in a separate room for two weeks. I was aware of the medical notion of birth and birth outcomes, but I couldn't go against the tradition. I pondered what if something bad happens to my baby. Following common practice was the best option for me to protect the baby from the cultural risks. Suntali

Suntali's experience suggests an opportunity exists for a collaborative model of childbirth to ensure physical and cultural safety to women living in the remote, rural and cross-cultural settings. Several forms of negotiation occurred in deciding the place of birth which allowed women to act in a way that maintained their culture, tradition and spiritual practices and led to the positive experiences. These examples demonstrate the possibility of negotiating different perspectives in a cross-cultural context to minimise risk and promote safety during childbirth.

The examples of negotiation with medical setting to maintain traditions and spirituality shared in other studies [11, 12] did not occur for these remote mountain women; rather they negotiated the birthing place choosing either the outside corner or the adjoining room of the house and only occasionally a health institution to replace the Goth. But all women followed the pollution practice during their postnatal days. This reflected their strong agency to transform the social structure according to the knowledge of constructing risk knowledge.

Remote mountain women were social actors which Giddens [13] discusses in his theory of structuration. These women were actively involved in recreating cultural values, traditional practice and spiritual beliefs in their childbirth practice as a way of reinforcing their social structure. In this process, some women were maintaining continuity of the tradition of giving birth in the Goth while others were more concerned about not creating ritual pollution. Although Jordan [14, 15] and Davis Floyd [16] consider women as the owners of their childbirth experiences, the ownership of birthing experiences for these women came through the continuation of collective tradition. As a part of the reform process, some women expressed strong determination to continue with the pollution belief in best possible ways.

Whatever happens: accepting the conditions of childbirth

Kitzinger [9] highlights the significance of giving birth in natural settings to ensure women's control of their childbirth. Remote mountain women had the opportunity to experience childbirth within their village, but they did not have control over the deaths occurring during the birth. So, the issue of survival of mothers and babies remained a complex issue in this cultural setting. Although there was a negotiation in practice of giving birth in the Goth in some women's experiences, their construction of knowledge about childbirth pollution did not allow them to go inside the house during the postnatal days.

Not all women had the same perceptions of childbirth but for most childbirth is a normal and recurring event in their everyday life routines. Considering childbirth as a normal part of everyday life events insulated women from medical influence over birth experiences. Despite the death of a newborn, some women accepted a spiritual understanding of birth and death and maintained the traditions.

Prema's account provides understanding of this perception of childbirth and related deaths.

> I am giving birth this month. I lost my previous baby boy nine months after the birth. I have three children; they are all girls. I hope this one is a boy. I don't know why my previous son died but we can't be happy only with these three daughters. I have never been to the hospital. I have never had any check-up. I have never had any problems giving birth. Who knows what happens? It isn't in our control. It is in God's hand. The baby will come, and they will go if the God wants. We can't stop them from dying. We just need to accept the reality – whatever happens during or after the birth – happens anyway. Prema

The inability to control the outcome of childbirth is a critical juncture in which women tend to simply accept the circumstances of their life. Getting pregnant and giving birth are unavoidable and continuous tasks for mountain women, and deaths are not something any available measures that can reliably prevent.

> Getting pregnant and giving birth is part of our life. There is nothing unusual about it. Women should get pregnant and give birth, it is given. What do we

do if we don't get pregnant and give birth? We get married, get pregnant and give birth. This is part of our life. I must work hard to feed the family. This is making me weaker, but these little children cannot work. What can I do? I can't avoid being pregnant and I can't stop working. I think we women are born to work and to give birth. Dolma

For all women, childbirth is a special experience but the meaning of giving birth differs in different contexts. For Dolma, marriage, pregnancy and childbirth are part of life and women should be able to manage without impacting the other tasks that family expect them to perform every day.

Jitu described childbirth as an ordinary naturally occurring event.

There is nothing different in giving birth. Giving birth to a child is always the same experience. The pain we experience during the birth is also the same. I didn't feel any difference about giving birth. It happened to be the same way all the time. This time as well, the baby came easily. I didn't have to experience a long pain. A slight pain started in the evening and I went to the room. By midnight, the pain gradually increased. The next morning, baby was out. I didn't have to call anyone for help. This is how I have been giving birth every time. I have never experienced any problems. Giving birth has always been easy task to me. Jitu

For these mountain women, experiencing pain was an expected part of the process of giving birth. The ability to give birth without experiencing any problems requiring external assistance was a satisfying experience for many women. However, some women were concerned about problems that had occurred while giving birth.

Laxmi is wondering why a problem occurred in her recent birth experience.

I didn't know anything about giving birth the first time, so I didn't have any fear. In God's favour, it all went well. Then only I knew how difficult or easy giving birth to a baby is. It hadn't been difficult giving birth to the previous babies. It happened normally. But this time, I don't know why there was bleeding before the baby. Family took me to the hospital. I still think that I should've been fine to give birth at home with my mother-in-law. Laxmi

Women seek medical help for only those problems which are not possible to manage at home. Going to hospital is a last resort for many women when they experience problems while giving birth. The belief that God plays an important role in minimising childbirth problems is still a strong perspective. Allowing women to seek social and family support while seeking medical care to manage problems could be a better way.

Changing ideas which challenge gender social expectations of childbirth as an essential everyday life task in the younger generation confronted some older women. Juna expressed her reservations about birth control.

> We get pregnant as many times as it comes and out body copes. We give birth as many times as the baby comes. We don't have any problems in doing so, as this is what we think women are supposed to do. These days, they [the younger generation] have stopped being pregnant [She indicates the use of family planning methods to control pregnancy]. You see they are going through so many problems while giving birth. They shouldn't try to stop the thing [indicating pregnancy] that is given by God. I will keep getting pregnant and giving birth until the God gives me that power. Juna

For Juna, childbirth is a spiritual event controlled by the wishes of God. In her view, attempting to act against the concept of childbirth as a natural phenomenon results in negative experiences. Conforming to spiritual, social and cultural expectations is important in protecting against the risks of death or illness associated with childbirth.

Walsh [17] notes that once we understand the central role of spirituality in childbirth, we can develop a better sense of why women do not adopt medical approaches. In this scenario, deaths continue without any medical interventions. Women consider birth and death as spiritual events. Some women shared their grief at multiple loss experiences.

Toli found it hard to accept the loss of babies as a natural event.

> During the cropping and harvesting season, women even give birth in the farm field. They use whatever is available around there while giving birth. Indeed, this isn't in our hands to make sure whether the mother or the baby will die or stay alive. But we can't happily accept the loss of the babies either. We like babies staying alive. It is hard. Toli

Unlike many others, Toli was reluctant to accept the losses as a normal part of childbirth. This provides an opportunity to develop interventions to promote survival of mothers and babies in the mountains. No women want to experience bad birth outcomes but how we can best support them to achieve positive childbirth experiences within their socio-cultural context is a critical matter.

Eckermann [12] and Liamputtong [18] provide examples of engagement with medicine in order to continue childbirth traditions and culture to maximise the safety. For the remote mountain women, similar engagement is possible without making them leave their preferred settings for childbirth to address the potential risks to mother and babies. This requires mutual negotiation as the current understanding of the risks as framed by cultural and medical paradigms is contradictory.

Sani, an older generation mother-in-law, raised the difference between knowledge frameworks.

> Back in our days, there wasn't a tradition of going to hospital. We didn't even have any health workers. These days they say [health workers and media] that pregnant women shouldn't be working hard and carrying heavy loads. It was different in our day. We believe continuing working helps to make our

body stronger and to give birth easily. During my daughter's turn, I was carrying wood for the whole day, maybe ten trips from the mountain. I milked five buffalos that evening, and I gave birth. I was by myself at home. My mother-in-law came and gave me a hand with the birth. Sani

The opposition of traditional knowledge and medical knowledge about work during pregnancy is another factor that women have found difficult to navigate while making decisions about their practices. The medical discourse challenged the belief that continuing everyday work facilitates the childbirth process and insisted women to avoid heavy loads and take enough rest during pregnancy. These women are not yet convinced by the information provided by the health workers as childbirth has always occurred as part of their daily work routines.

Rama spoke about how differences between social and medical expectations put women in a complex situation when making choices about childbirth.

In the village, people say that it depends on luck to have better childbirth experiences. Whatever happens is due to luck, you know fortune – yes it depends how fortunate you are. People didn't like me going to the hospital, as they think I am acting against the social norms and practice. The older women in the village talk about their childbirth experiences and say that they did all the work without any special consideration during their pregnancy. They expect us to do the same. They question any woman that goes to hospital for a check-up or to give birth. It isn't easy. So, we must accept whatever comes our way. This is like living at the end of dark tunnel. Rama

Situations like this make the information women receive about care required during pregnancy or childbirth become meaningless. Women remain powerless to challenge culture norms and handle the impact on them of acting against social expectations. The difference between generations in understanding childbirth makes it difficult for younger women to accept medical care.

These beliefs affirm that childbirth in mountain villages is an ongoing, natural and easy event that occurs as a normal part of their everyday life. The interaction of culture, spiritual beliefs and tradition in determining the survival of newborn babies revealed by these stories opens the possibility of the socio-cultural and medical paradigm working together. It is important to note that, given the gap in understanding between cultural and medical knowledge of risk is significant, the stories shared by women show the effectiveness of managing childbirth problems in a collaborative way. This evidence could facilitate the development of a new model of cross-cultural care for women without compromising their perception of safety in the institutional settings.

Oakley [19] and Kitzinger [9] point out that the concept of childbirth as a normal socio-cultural event and posed concern how western society has shifted this to a medicalised event. Brunson [20] found a similar shift happening among urban women in Nepal. Unlike this shifting, remote mountain women described childbirth as a normal and ongoing task by accepting their everyday context as a social expectation. As Douglas [21] highlights how medicine often blames culture for causing high maternal and newborn deaths, the similar blame was made against the family for causing maternal and newborn deaths in the village. Young [22] writes that community people do not trust others who they do not know well. This was evident when women preferred seeking help from Traditional Faith Healers in the village and denied medical help when they experience problems. Their strong connection to faith and tradition created a situation of certainties and uncertainties of maternal and newborn survival.

Will survive or die: certainty and uncertainty of birth outcomes

An individual's decision about their actions is based on knowledge of risk and uncertainties [23]. Women who linked their worry to the uncertainties of outcomes did not make any decisions to change their birthing practice. The feeling of uncertainty did not influence the change in cultural beliefs and traditional practices of giving birth. They expressed the same level of trust in God who could be helpful to deal with associated uncertainties and ensure positive outcomes. This belief in spiritual power provided them with a safe boundary to remain within their socio-cultural setting.

While childbirth was taken to be a part of the events of everyday life, the reality of its certainties and uncertainties emerged in the women's stories. On the one hand, women maintain that God controls the birth, survival and death. On the other hand, women were anxious when they could not be sure of survival or death. Those who had experienced perinatal and neonatal losses expressed this dilemma. As experiences are a source of knowledge [24], certainty is in the hope for survival of the mother and her babies and uncertainty is represented by the threat of death.

Pema and her husband spoke together to explain the notion of uncertainties.

> We are worried about this baby. We lost our previous child on the ninth day of birth. You know, it was a son [with an emphasis]. This time we don't know what is going to happen. We hope that the birth will go in a good way. We don't expect anything to turn another way. We are hoping this will be a son too. What can we do if God wants the things to happen the other way? We can't do anything about that, so we just need to wait and see. Pema and her husband

In the context of uncertainty, while maintaining hope they will not experience another loss, the faith that it is God that determines survival remains strong for this couple. A similar experience of loss prompted Toli to seek medical care in the hope of avoiding the risk of losing a baby again, but she did not find it helpful.

> I gave birth to twins last time, but they died within 10 days. They turned yellow; I think they had jaundice. Because of that experience, I was anxious about the condition of the baby this time. So, I went to the hospital for a

check-up, but I did not get any help. They didn't even check me well. They couldn't tell me whether the baby is well or not. I came back not knowing how my unborn baby is. I hope the God will help me to go through this well and I will have a baby alive. Toli

The lack of faith in medical care is evident here when the services that Toli received failed to meet her expectations. This experience reaffirmed her spiritual understanding of safety in which God is the only hope in preventing death. The lack of certainty of the outcome of a birth that concerned these families remained unresolved. There is no way to ensure survival.

For these women, the social obligation to produce children is another reason that exacerbates the uncertainty of birth outcomes. There was an expectation that a married woman should get pregnant and give birth, as soon as possible.

Sunita mentioned how she had to get pregnant even when she did not feel ready or safe for it.

I am feeling lonely, worried and helpless. I didn't want to get pregnant this early, but I couldn't avoid it. I wanted to terminate it but he [husband] told me I must continue it. I am so anxious about it. Though I live within laws, no one listens to me or cares about my feelings. I am feeling sick day by day. I have some sorts of fear as I don't know what giving birth is like. I am worried about the things that can happen during and after the birth. I think I might die while giving birth. But honestly, I am not worried about dying. Now, I have no more wish to live this way. Sunita

Sunita's experiences stress the psychological impacts of pregnancy in a complex situation in which she had no control over decisions involving her fertility. Rather, she conformed to the expectations and decisions made by her husband. The fear and uncertainty about survival, the feeling of helplessness and lack of emotional support during pregnancy raised in Sunita's account are important aspects to consider in making childbirth a safe and satisfying experience for women. It is unacceptable that women feel that a pregnancy can end their life or that they are better off dying than living in such difficult circumstances. These issues must be addressed so that women have choices and the power to make decisions about when they would like to get pregnant and how they want to experience childbirth.

When women learnt about the possible problems that could occur before, during or after childbirth, they were anxious. Rita expressed her worries.

I am so upset. Since he [husband] left, I am feeling helpless. I am worried about giving birth. I know many problems could happen while giving birth. There are other people supporting me emotionally, but I miss my husband. Not having him around doesn't feel the same. I am worried about so many things. I am thinking all the time how will this birth take place? Oh God, I hope everything goes well. I just can't stop thinking about it and it has been stressful lately. Rita

Rita's story makes clear the nature of support that women want during childbirth. When women were not able to get the support they need, it created fear, distress and feelings of insecurity. As a result, women lack confidence and are not certain about their capacity to make childbirth a safe and happy experience. While the spiritual significance of childbirth provided cultural security to women, it also highlighted a sense of uncertainty regarding the survival of mother and baby.

Kiru spoke about the inherent uncertainties of surviving childbirth.

> Who knows what is going to happen? Who knows whether the baby will come alive or die? Who knows whether I will survive or die in giving birth? Nobody knows what will happen. Only God knows what is going to happen. Last time I felt dead, but luckily, I survived. Kiru

The fact that birth and death was beyond human control consistently appeared in the stories that women shared has significance in considering ways to minimise threats to maternal and newborn survival in complex social settings. When women experienced problems either during the pregnancy or during childbirth, they started pondering about how these problems could be minimised in subsequent experiences.

Manu spoke about that worry.

> I am feeling very weak [kamjor] this time. I wasn't like this before. I was strong. My belly is also very big. I don't know why it is big. It wasn't like that before. Sometimes they said (in radio), the baby can come earlier. None of my babies came early before. I don't know what will happen this time. Because of God's choice, I didn't have any problem up until now. This time, I am a bit worried. Manu

These stories illustrate the uncertain emotional state of women when their expectations based on previous birth experiences were not met or their needs to be well prepared for giving birth were not supported. The knowledge of childbirth that women developed through experience enabled them to identify some problems and that prompted some women to seek additional help. However, in most cases, knowledge of problems related to childbirth likely to occur did not change their practice but simply added to the stress of uncertainty.

There is an opposition in understanding of adverse birth outcomes between the socio-cultural and the medical perspective. While the women linked childbirth problems and the ultimate outcome of the birth to the choice of "God," medical doctors held the family responsible for not taking appropriate actions to manage problems which resulted in the death of a mother.

> One case of maternal death happened this year in the hospital. It was a festival time and people were celebrating in the village. She gave birth at home and had her placenta stuck inside. She bled and bled and bled. She had lots of bleeding. No one noticed until she went into shock. Her family didn't bring

her to the hospital on time. It was the last minute by the time she reached hospital. We tried to resuscitate her, but it was too late. She died. Medical doctor

The medical discourse has confidence in the capacity of clinical interventions to save lives of mothers and babies in institutional settings and would like women to come to hospital to give birth. In the circumstances where greater emphasis is given on spiritual safety, it is difficult to find the best solution for promoting maternal and newborn survival. The medical model of childbirth is not attractive to women when it does not acknowledge and incorporate important aspects of culture, tradition and spiritual practice.

These stories further illustrate the place of traditional healing practices in managing childbirth problems. Women tend to trust the local traditional faith healer ability to manage problems.

> When women give birth at Goth and the placenta normally stuck inside. They don't go to hospital or call a health worker to get help. Instead, they consult the Dhami and Jhankri [two different types of Traditional Faith Healers] for a spiritual healing process. Most of the time, they call me for help. I help them during such conditions. I have asked them to go to hospital, but they don't want to do that. They trust us [Dhami and Jhankri] and I think it is my duty to help them. Traditional faith healer

Women's childbirth experiences embed with faith regarding traditional childbirth knowledge and support. This has been important for women to create a sense of certainty regarding birth outcomes. Their faith in the traditional healing process to manage childbirth problems is an important aspect that needs consideration to understand the social context of women's decisions. Because of their faith, women give greater value to traditional knowledge.

A local politician explained this emphasis on traditional knowledge.

> Still, there is strong cultural belief and traditional practices in the village where people trust more in Traditional Faith Healers for example Dhami and Jhankri during the sickness [this refers to childbirth related problems as well]. There are high numbers of childbirth related deaths in the village. Only yesterday, two babies died. Local politician

The gap in understanding between the medical and cultural view of childbirth makes it challenging to address the factors causing maternal and newborn deaths in remote mountain villages. As women value traditional knowledge more than medical knowledge, they are unlikely to be attracted to medical care. Certainly, these women's childbirth experiences induce feelings of both certainty and uncertainty around potential birth outcomes. Most women felt that it was only supernatural power which would determine safe birth outcomes. This spiritual belief informed their practices with the idea that God controls birth and death. According to this belief, acting against God led to negative experiences. For these women, controlling desired birth outcomes is impossible, as it is determined by God, based on their actions.

Women indicate that the paradigm of risk posited by medical knowledge holds cultural and spiritual practices responsible for maternal and newborn deaths, whereas other women see medical interventions as threats to childbirth safety. Consequently, faith in medical care is compromised and women prefer traditional healing to manage childbirth problems. Although women were worried about uncertain outcomes, it did not change their beliefs or practices which contain expectations that the spiritual healing process will prevent deaths and promote the chances of survival. Consequently, women were prepared to accept whatever outcome occurred and accepted death as an inevitable part of childbirth. The only viable option is to create services that meet the cultural and spiritual needs of women while also ensuring improved survival of mothers and babies.

Sickle or blade: a dilemma of ensuring safety

The practice of using the sickle or blade for cutting the newborn cord is common in mountain villages of Nepal. This cord cutting practice creates the risk of infection [25–27] although some see it as associated with higher rates of newborn survival. A randomised controlled trial conducted in a rural Nepal identified that safe cord cutting practice could prevent the deaths of newborn babies [28]. There is not enough evidence to confirm whether the traditional cord cutting practice results in higher numbers of newborn deaths in the mountain. Using sickles or blades to cut the cord is a common practice that medical professionals identify as a source of neonatal infections.

The sickle is a tool generally used for cutting vegetables or grass which women have easy access to during childbirth. The sickle has a large sharp blade with a short handle that women frequently use to cut the cord of newborn babies. Some women use a razor instead – typically a razor used for shaving by men. Women were not yet aware of the problems that the use of the sickle or blade can cause for newborn survival.

Pema explained how cord cutting was done with her baby.

> We put the cord of the baby on timber and we cut the cord using a sickle or whatever is available at that time. After cutting the cord, we put some warm mustard oil on the Navi [umbilicus]. We leave the cord open without tying. Pema

The cord cutting practice described here is consistent with other studies which highlighted the practice as posing a risk of causing newborn infections and neonatal death [25–27, 29].

Lashi used the similar cord cutting practice but was not sure why her baby fell sick.

> Aunty found a sickle on the ceiling and used that to cut the cord of the baby. She left the cord open, but I don't remember whether she put anything on

it [umbilicus] after. Nothing wrong happened after the birth, but now he is very sick. He had a fever for the last three days. I don't know what caused the fever. Lashi

An association between this cord cutting practice and neonatal infections has been reported in previous studies [30, 31]. There has been no research conducted in the mountain villages to examine the correlation between the cord cutting practices and neonatal infections or deaths. Cord cutting practices could be one of the factors impacting newborn survival; however, it is still difficult to be certain what is causing the sickness and deaths of the newborn babies in these villages.

The use of a new blade could reduce the chance of newborn infection [25]. It was encouraged in the newborn care training delivered by the DHO that Manu had the opportunity to attend in her role as FCHV. However, she did not have a new blade during her own birth and had no options to use other measures.

> I used a blade to cut the cord of my previous baby, an old blade because I couldn't find the new one. I tied the cord with string, the same string we use to sew the cloth. I made two knots and tied in two places. They told us during the training that we should make tight two knots. I did so. They also said to use a new blade and boiled string. But I didn't do that. I had no one to help me to do all that during the birth. Manu

This study revealed that women's management of risk does not conform with the medical explanation of what actions to take for safe childbirth outcomes. The information about risks and ways of mitigating those risks can only be effective in practice if women have access to the resources and services within the village at the time of childbirth. Lacking these resources results in greater reliance on the safety provided by spiritual practices to promote the survival of the baby.

Urgen was another FCHV from the village that attended the same training provided by the DHO. She spoke about the complexities of maintaining medical and spiritual safety to ensure survival.

> They [health workers] told us during the training that we need to use a safe delivery kit during childbirth. But they didn't give any kits to bring home. How can we get the kit to use if they don't provide it to us? We can't get it in the village. My mother always cut the cord with a sickle. This time also we will do the same. If the baby is going to die, we can't stop it happening anyway. It is all God's wishes. Urgen

A study conducted in Nepal found that the use of a safe birthing kit (which usually includes a sterile blade) is beneficial in preventing umbilical cord infection [32]. However, women in this study revealed the difficulties in creating knowledge around risk and in identifying the causes of newborn deaths. This shows a compromised intervention in cord cutting practice which further illustrates how traditional knowledge is maintained to continue childbirth traditions in practice. The presentation of a traditional practice as risky, which the women see as normal, creates another difficulty in ensuring newborn survival. Nevertheless, there is a possibility of changing the practice through a development of an ongoing health initiative which includes making resources and services available to women locally.

Douglas [21, 33] notes that an individual's understanding of circumstances influences their way of perceiving and constructing safety, which is consistent with the experiences of remote mountain women. Most women were not aware of the risks; however, they were aware of what contributed to make their childbirth experiences positive and satisfying. Their traditional knowledge was important and resulted in their trust and confidence to continue the tradition and cultural practices. As Lupton [34] points out, types of knowledge, whether traditional or medical, influence childbirth practices. Some women, who were aware of the medical risks, were keen to use medical services. But others were concerned that the impacts can arise from not following their traditions and spirituality. Consistent with Douglas [21], all the women were committed to maintain the culture, tradition and spirituality to ensure childbirth safety.

Conclusion

The medical model considers childbirth as a physiological event; however, remote mountain women shaped their birth experiences by their underpinning socio-cultural constructs and practices. Women feel comfortable to be within their socio-cultural circumstances while giving birth which has been significant to enhance their perception of safety and women made best arrangements to maintain the childbirth tradition. Women felt threatened while giving birth in the institutional environment and the determination to stay within the community to give birth became stronger even when the survival of mother or babies are uncertain. This indicates the value that culture, tradition, spirituality, belief system, local knowledge and social norms play is shaping the childbirth practice in cross-cultural communities and how this contributes to create a sense of safety for birthing women and their respective society.

Nevertheless, we cannot deny the economic and social costs of preventable maternal and newborn deaths occurring in these remote communities, important though it is to acknowledge the implications of maintaining cultural and emotional safety of women during pregnancy, childbirth and postnatal periods. Without an attempt to understand and give attention to the social, economic and cultural environment that women give birth to, improving the experiences and childbirth outcomes may take longer than expected. Taking lived experiences of these women into the account, we must respect the socio-cultural circumstances of women while designing and providing services to enable safe, empowering and satisfying childbirth experiences to all women.

References

1   Douglas, M., *Purity and danger [1966]*. 1991: Routledge, London.
2   Wallerstein, N., *Empowerment to reduce health disparities*. Scandinavian Journal of Public Health, 2002. **30**(59): p. 72–77.

3   Wagle, R.R., S. Sabroe, and B.B. Nielsen, *Socioeconomic and physical distance to the maternity hospital as predictors for place of delivery: An observation study from Nepal.* BMC Pregnancy and Childbirth, 2004. **4**(1): p. 8.

4   Triandis, H.C., et al., *Individualism and collectivism: Cross-cultural perspectives on self-ingroup relationships.* Journal of Personality and Social Psychology, 1988. **54**(2): p. 323.

5   Fox, B. and D. Worts, *Revisiting the critique of medicalized childbirth: A contribution to the sociology of birth.* Gender and Society, 1999. **13**(3): p. 326–346.

6   Labonte, R., *Heart health inequalities in Canada: Modules, theory and planning.* Health Promotion International, 1992. **7**(2): p. 119–128.

7   Oakley, A., *Women confined: Towards a sociology of childbirth.* 1980: Schocken, New York.

8   Regmi, K., R. Smart, and J. Kottler, *Understanding gender and power dynamics within the family: a qualitative study of Nepali women's experience.* Australian and New Zealand Journal of Family Therapy, 2010. **31**(2): p. 191–201.

9   Kitzinger, S., *Some cultural perspectives of birth.* British Journal of Midwifery, 2000. **8**(12): p. 746–750.

10 Callister, L.C., S. Semenic, and J.C. Foster, *Cultural and spiritual meanings of childbirth: Orthodox Jewish and Mormon women.* Journal of Holistic Nursing, 1999. **17**(3): p. 280–295.

11 Rice, P.L. and J. Lumley, *Childbirth and soul loss: The case of a Hmong woman.* Medical Journal of Australia, 1994. **160**(9): p. 577–578.

12 Eckermann, L., *Finding a 'safe' place on the risk continuum: A case study of pregnancy and birthing in Lao PDR.* Health Sociology Review, 2006. **15**(4): p. 374–386.

13 Giddens, A., *The constitution of society: Outline of the theory of structuration.* 1984: University of California Press, Oakland.

14 Jordan, B., *Birth in four cultures: A cross-cultural investigation of childbirth in Yucatan, Holland, Sweden and the United States.* 1978: Waveland Press, Long Grove.

15 Jordan, B., *Birth in four cultures: A cross-cultural investigation of childbirth in Yucatan, Holland, Sweden, and the United States.* 1992: Waveland Press, Long Grove.

16 Davis-Floyd, R.E. and C.F. Sargent, *Childbirth and authoritative knowledge: Cross-cultural perspectives.* 1997: University of California Press, Oakland.

17 Walsh, D.J., *Childbirth embodiment: Problematic aspects of current understandings.* Sociology of Health and Illness, 2010. **32**(3): p. 486–501.

18 Liamputtong, P., Pregnancy, childbirth and traditional beliefs and practices in Chiang Mai, Northern Thailand, in *Childbirth across cultures.* 2009: Springer. p. 175–184.

19 Oakley, A., *Childbirth practice should take women's wishes into account.* BMJ: British Medical Journal, 1996. **313**(7071): p. 1557.

20 Brunson, J., *Confronting maternal mortality, controlling birth in Nepal: The gendered politics of receiving biomedical care at birth.* Social Science and Medicine, 2010. **71**(10): p. 1719–1727.

21 Douglas, M., *Risk and Blame: An analysis of concepts of pollution and taboo.* 1992: Routledge, London.

22 Young, I.M., *Five faces of oppression. Rethinking power.* 2014: State University of New York Press, New York.

23 Kaphle, S., H. Hancock, and L.A. Newman, *Childbirth traditions and cultural perceptions of safety in Nepal: Critical spaces to ensure the survival of mothers and newborns in remote mountain villages.* Midwifery, 2013. **29**(10): p. 1173–1181.

24 Kolbe, D.A., *Experiential learning: Experience as the source of learning and development.* 2014: Pearson Education, New York.

25   Mullany, L.C., et al., *Risk factors for umbilical cord infection among newborn of southern Nepal.* American Journal of Epidemiology, 2007. **165**(2): p. 203–211.

26   Mullany, L.C., et al., *Topical applications of chlorhexidine to the umbilical cord for prevention of omphalitis and neonatal mortality in southern Nepal: A community-based, cluster-randomised trial.* The Lancet, 2006. **367**(9514): p. 910–918.

27   Mullany, L.C., et al., *Traditional massage of newborns in Nepal: Implications for trials of improved practice.* Journal of Tropical Paediatrics, 2005. **51**(2): p. 82–86.

28   Osrin, D., et al., *Cross sectional, community based study of care of newborn infants in Nepal.* British Medical Journal, 2002. **325**(7372): p. 1063.

29   Sreeramareddy, C.T., et al., *Home delivery and newborn care practices among urban women in western Nepal: A questionnaire survey.* BMC Pregnancy and Childbirth, 2006. **6**(1): p. 27.

30   Liljestrand, J., *Reducing perinatal and maternal mortality in the world: The major challenges.* British Journal of Obstetrics and Gynaecology, 1999. **106**(9): p. 877.

31   Stoll, B.J., *The global impact of neonatal infection.* Clinics in Perinatology, 1997. **24**(1): p. 1–21.

32   Rhee, V., et al., *Maternal and birth attendant hand washing and neonatal mortality in southern Nepal.* Archives of Paediatrics and Adolescent Medicine, 2008. **162**(7): p. 603–608.

33   Douglas, M., *Purity and danger: An analysis of conception of body and pollution.* 1991: Routledge, London.

34   Lupton, D., *Risk and sociocultural theory: New directions and perspectives.* 1999: Cambridge University Press, Cambridge.

5 Women, family members and significant others

Paradox of power

Introduction

"Who do you live with currently, Rita Sister?" I began.

"I live with my in-laws as my husband has gone overseas and my mother died when I was only 10 years old," she responded.

"Do you find this living arrangement hard?"

"They don't understand me, and I need to do whatever they say. I miss my mother a lot. If she were alive it would be much easier to live with her. I am an educated woman, yet I can't make any decisions. My in-laws are traditional, and they don't listen to me. Unlike most men, my husband is supportive and understanding, but not having him around makes things even harder and I have no options to go anywhere now," she continued.

"What about others in the village?"

The majority are conservative and want us to do things the way they did in the past. Everyone thinks they are right in their own way. It is frustrating and upsetting at the same time." Rita became emotional at this point.

"What about your experience of antenatal visits?" I changed the topic.

"They [health workers] usually do the checks, do injections needed and tell us when the next visit is due. They ask us to go to hospital to give birth or in an emergency. That is kind of it." She paused.

The socio-cultural conditions in which women give birth provide a deeper understanding of the core values of a society [1, 2]. From a social-constructionist and critical-feminist point of view, it is important to consider social norms, expectations, interactions and relationships while making the meaning of childbirth [3]. This perspective emphasises the criticality of women having control of their experiences in promoting safety and survival during childbirth [4]. Women's experiences of childbirth are influenced by various patterns of relationship both within and outside household hierarchies where negotiation and trust play important roles in determining how childbirth is viewed and experienced within their social circumstances. Based on the experiences shared by the women, the influence of these relationships on childbirth experiences are explored through two lenses – one relating to their status as women, and the other in respect of the care and support provided to women.

Who are we? Social roles and positioning of women

> Men in this village ignore women and don't bother about household chores. They are happy drinking Chyang [traditional alcoholic drink] and talking nonsense. Women stay at home doing all the work. Men spend money to entertain themselves. Why shouldn't they take responsibility for the family? I am struggling to feed these children. It is always the same for women: the same household chores, taking care of children, getting pregnant and giving birth. Men don't understand our problems. He [husband] left home early this morning; maybe he is drinking somewhere with other men. He doesn't even worry about our sick child. How can he take care of me if he doesn't care of his children? Women are like shoes on their feet. The health worker asked my husband to use family planning; he didn't listen. Instead, he came home and said to me that he will go to India if I ask him to have a vasectomy or stop having sex. My body is getting weaker day by day and he doesn't understand it. Villagers don't understand either. They just tease me for getting pregnant at this age [indicating older age]. It is hard for me to cope everything. Urgen

Gender is a culturally defined status marker for differences in power relationships and plays a crucial role in childbirth decisions [5–8]. Understanding gender, what it means to be a man and a woman can often take paradoxical forms [9]. In Nepalese society, tensions sometimes emerge as gender-based understandings are adapted and renegotiated by men and women as they attempt to understand their roles [10]. This tension is observed in the childbirth experiences of remote mountain women. As most women hold a subordinate status in families with structural role differences [11], this influence of power unfolds in a similar way in how women experience childbirth.

Although women accepted the support provided by family members and others during childbirth, they also experienced differences in many aspects of their experience. Structural power differences within the household and social expectations in relationships became crucial components in defining a woman's role. Thus, women were mostly involved in domestic and agricultural chores. It appeared that maintaining social expectations was the priority for most women as this is how their position was constructed within the society.

Jitu was concerned about the amount of work she was doing during her early postnatal days.

> He [husband] asked me to prepare things [herbal medicinal drinks] to treat our sick cow. I had to do that before cooking something for myself to eat. I have too much work to do every day. No one in the family will do it [work] or help me to finish chores if I don't. Our men don't do any work. I need to manage all the chores and look after the baby. Jitu

Women's needs were accorded the lowest priority even in the critical period after childbirth. Getting household chores done was put ahead of taking care of the baby or their own health. Hence, most women accepted their socially defined roles and introduced themselves as working women. Generally, they were involved in the bearing and rearing of children, performing household chores, farming, carrying food from the market, walking long distances to collect water and involvement in other community activities. For women, continuing these tasks was mandatory. There was a perception that continuing this work throughout pregnancy would facilitate a normal birth. When women were unable to continue the same amount of work during pregnancy, it raised concerns about whether the birth would occur in a normal manner or not.

Manu shared her worries.

> In the village, we [women] need to work hard. We are the ones to manage all work, inside or outside the house. If we don't work, everyone [in the family] will die of hunger. The men take no stress about the work or the hardships of feeding the family. It is women's work. It is different, as we are women. I did all the work throughout my pregnancies – until the time of giving birth. I don't feel that I have the strength anymore. I can't work in the same capacity as I used to do before. I may not be able to give birth normally this time because I haven't been working enough and I lost my strengths. Manu

Where the power difference and gendered division of tasks was a socially accepted construct, women questioned why men did not take responsibility for household chores. The role of women as workers within and outside the household did not change during pregnancy but not being able to physically maintain that role resulted in emotional threats. This raises further questions about the gendered concept of work and its impacts on childbirth in these remote settings. The household responsibilities performed by women were not economically counted or acknowledged. Historically, the Hindu religion assigns women into the category of performing household chores including childbearing and rearing tasks [12]. These duties were prescribed for women, and thus are unavoidable.

Rima spoke about these sanctioned duties.

> Women are different to men. We [women] are supposed to be occupied with household chores. It is not nice for women to run a poorly managed household or spend time watching television or going outside for entertainment. We are expected to remain inside the household boundaries. We should maintain our Dharma [duties] being women. Rima

Focusing on what women and men do raises questions of social positioning and the division of labour with complex interactions to define roles within or outside households. This complexity is apparent for these women, as their duties were not limited to the domestic sphere or to religious codes and all women have the same level of responsibilities to perform every day.

Toli talked about the work women do outside their domestic chores.

> We usually go to Lek [high-altitude farmland] during the cropping season. I was there [at Lek] a week before I gave birth. It is seven to eight hours walk from this village to the farming area. Others have already gone to start

cropping potatoes and barley. I need to go to Lek as early as possible, otherwise we won't get good potatoes. If I don't go early, no one else in the family
will go and do it. This is the task for me to complete. Toli

Panter-Brick [13] wrote about his observations of Nepali women in the mountains
who walked long distances during pregnancy carrying a baby on their back. I have
seen some women putting their baby to one side under a temporary shelter while
working in the fields. This is somehow better than leaving a newborn away from
their mother for a full day but still raises concerns about their safety during the
early postnatal period. Normally, women worked long hours.
    Tolma talked about her everyday routine.

> You want to know about my work. It is not like the work you do in the city.
> My day starts with the rooster's first call. The water tap isn't close to our
> house. I need to bring water for household use – generally four times every
> day; each trip takes about 20 minutes. I cook for the children and feed them.
> I have some goats and cows in the house. I need to take care of them as well.
> I prepare snacks for the children and for the people working with me in the
> field. I go to the field after finishing the household chores in the morning. In
> the field, what we crop follows the seasons. Now, it is the season for wheat,
> barley and potatoes. Basically, these are the only thing we could grow in our
> mountains. We all are preparing the soil now. Every day is a busy day. I return
> home only towards the late evening. Tolma

Unlike women, men were involved in direct income activities which did not
require undertaking household or agricultural work.
    Dolma talked about the work that men generally perform in the village.

> Our [women's] work is different to their [men's] work. Men are more con-
> cerned with business, entertainment, travel and other income. They usually
> travel to different places for their business and other activities. We don't even
> know what they actually do when they are away for business. We [women]
> need to be involved in household chores and farming. Isn't that what a woman
> is supposed to be doing anyway? This is how we have seen the work divided
> between men and women. Why would a husband do household chores? It
> wouldn't suit men to do women's work. Dolma

Traditionally defined gender roles influence the practice whereby men have significantly lighter workloads than women [14]. Gendered social norms shape the
views of women with the consensus being to continue with the regular tasks in order
to adhere to social expectations. The roles of men as breadwinners and women as
household managers are widely accepted social roles [15–18]. This gendered division of labour has resulted in women having a higher burden of household tasks.
Despite attempts made towards gender equity in Nepal, it is undeniable that economic, social and cultural inequalities exist [19]. While women play the central

role in the subsistence of the family, gendered obligations constructed by society remain a challenge when it comes to sexuality, reproduction and childbirth. In this social environment, some women felt the continued burden of pregnancy and childbirth. Sadly, they were not able to resist these expectations.

Hira mentioned the complexities from her perspective.

> It would've been better if we [women] didn't need to give birth so many times. What can we do? We must give birth again and again. If I tell my husband that I don't want to get pregnant, he will certainly find another wife. I have no choice. This is all about him, not me. I must be ready for it, stay quiet and follow his choice. Our [women's] life will continue like this. Hira

In a society which treats women as objects to serve the interests of men, the legitimacy of power sits with men and denies rights by creating further vulnerability for women. This puts pressure on women to obey the wishes of their husband without any consideration of their own interests or choices. This indicated a form of structural oppression existing in the marital relationship.

Pema shared similar frustrations.

> The life of a married woman is very hard in the village. Once we get married; the task is getting pregnant, giving birth, looking after children, following interests of husband and serving the family. Our men don't listen to the women. We can't say no to our husband. Pema

Most women felt unheard and powerless. The impact of unequal power relationships between men and women on their childbirth decisions led to the pressure of accepting pregnancy and childbirth as a continual routine for women. Yet they raised hopes for shared understanding that couples could develop to make appropriate decisions.

Urgen suggested one possibility for improving the status of women.

> If we give opportunities for girls' education; it would help to make their lives happier and easier. That is why I am sending them [her daughters and daughter-in-law] to school. I am hoping that they won't need to live like me – being a servant to the family. Men have made women's lives harder. Women can't say no to their husbands when they come and sleep [indicating sex] with them. Women can't ignore their husband's wishes. Unless men accept that they need to limit the number of children in their family and take care of their wife's body, the situation here will remain the same. So, we need to make our men aware first. Urgen

Education and awareness play an important role in developing supportive relationships between men and women. Urgen pointed out that educating women and creating awareness among men could enable social change whereby women are no longer voiceless or oppressed. Freire's [20] perspective on education creates awareness through subjective understanding of the conditions of the world and the conditions that shape them supports this view of social change in making childbirth decisions. Sadly, many men still think of childbirth as women's business. However, women were keen to experience equal sharing of workloads with mutual understanding in their relationship.

Kabita shared her view.

> I think it would be better if men share equal workloads with women. Having a shared understanding between husband and wife in issues relating to their lives would be helpful. It will be good if the couple [husband and wife] work together with mutual understanding. Kabita

A similar possibility for reducing the amount of domestic work that women do is through enlisting the understanding of family members has been discussed [21]. However, in a structural power relationship where women hold subordinate status, the authority of men over women impacted childbirth decisions making women unable to speak against the wishes of men. Consequently, the tasks of getting pregnant and giving birth become a part of everyday life routines for these women.

Nevertheless, the optimism shared by the women about improving their status through developing shared understandings and responsibilities between men and women signifies the possibility of creating a dialogue to construct negotiated understandings of gender at household and societal levels. This negotiated construct could enable women to make decisions about significant life events including childbirth.

Being together or apart: the crucial influence of relationships

In the hierarchical family structures of Nepal, women follow more traditional gender roles to meet social expectations and are often restricted in making childbirth decisions. In this social structure, the mother-in-law becomes the prime influence in deciding where and how to give birth. The mother-in-law's decision about childbirth is mostly supported by other family members. Occasionally, educated husbands interfere in decisions to ensure the safety of birth outcomes. Women spoke about how these relationships influenced their childbirth experiences.

Mother-in-law and daughter-in-law: a critical relationship

Women's status varies within the context of social structures, where their position as a mother-in-law holds a respected and powerful status [22]. This hierarchical structure allows mothers-in-law to exert power over their daughters-in-law [21]. Traditionally, girls were raised to be submissive in their status as a daughter-in-law and avoid speaking out against the family [23], a practice which can still be observed in Nepalese society. It is a common trend that when a married girl fails to be respectful to her in laws her parents are blamed, most specifically the mother. The influence of the significant power dynamics in this relationship was reflected in childbirth – with both positive and negative experiences.

Some relationships between mother-in-law and daughter-in-law were reciprocal with mutual respect, understanding and shared values. For example, Sumi (daughter-in-law) and Maina (mother-in-law) were able to develop a shared understanding.

Daughter-in-law Sumi mentioned how the support of her mother-in-law contributed to positive childbirth experiences.

> My mother-in-law was there with me all the time. She helped me to give birth. I didn't know anything about how to deal with these things. She did everything to me. I didn't need to worry about the baby either. This time we were planning to give birth at home, but the baby didn't come, and we went to the hospital. She [mother-in-law] came along and supported me. She is the one to look after me and the baby, which makes me feel happy. I feel lucky to have her. Sumi

This example of the supportive contribution of power in this relationship was linked with the respect and trust they were able to establish. This was further connected with the childbirth knowledge that the mother-in-law possessed in order to make the decision whether the woman needed medical help or not. Trusting in the decision made by her mother-in-law helped the woman feel safe and happy.

Mother-in-law Maina spoke about mutual trust and understanding in the relationship.

> Kanchi [the youngest daughter-in-law, Sumi] loves me and looks after me very well. I also love her and take care of her well. It isn't a one-sided coin; it must be two sided. I tried the same with my oldest daughter-in-law [Jethi] but she didn't listen and ignored me completely. Unlike us, she [Jethi] went to school and thinks she knows better. I am happy with Kanchi. We understand each other's pain and discomfort. I will let her have complete rest for a month. I won't ask her to do any hard work until two months (after the birth). I didn't have such a rest period during my time. Now, I realise that women giving birth need enough rest and better food. I will provide as much as I can for Kanchi. Maina

Exercising power and authority over a daughter-in-law by a mother-in-law is a customary practice in this hierarchical family structure and respect towards the mother-in-law is expected. However, a shift in power is possible in these critical relationships as some daughters-in-law were starting to make their own decisions about childbirth. Along with the influence of education, a generational gap in understanding created some tensions in the relationship.

The relationship between Hira (mother-in-law) and Laxmi (daughter-in-law) illustrates tensions in managing role expectations. The mother-in-law Hira spoke about the different nature of relationships she had with her daughters-in-law.

> In my time, I even had two pregnancies within a year. I took that burden. Now, I am a mother-in-law. I tell Jethi [Laxmi] to do light work, to eat better food

and to stay with me, so we share the comfort. I didn't get such an opportunity during my time. But I feel how important it is to support them before, during and after childbirth. Another daughter-in-law [Kanchi] does not respect me or follow my advice. Jethi will tell you that I am a good person in the village. If you talk to Kanchi, she will tell you that I am a bad person. She turns the other way if I see her by chance. She doesn't talk to me. For me both are equal, but I don't know why Kanchi reacts to me so differently. Hira

Daughter-in-law Laxmi confirmed the positive nature of their relationship.

My mother-in-law usually tells me to work less, eat well and maintain hygiene. I spend most of my time with her. We don't have any conflict or misunderstandings. She takes care of me very well. I think it needs to be two sided. Daughters-in-law should respect their mothers-in-law to ensure care and support in return. Sadly, for some this relationship is fraught. It doesn't have to be like that, they can get on well together. We are close and trust one other. She understands me well and I respect her. I trust her when she tells me what to do. Laxmi

Unlike positive relationships that contributed to enhancing safe childbirth experiences, relationships that lacked mutual understanding and trust resulted in confusion and conflict, which complicated the harmonious family values. A generational gap resulting from changing channels of information and knowledge created misunderstanding in these relationships.

Urgen was a mother-in-law and was living with her own mother. She talked about the changing nature of relationships.

My mother supported the birth of all the children. But my daughter-in-law doesn't share things with us [me and my mother]. She thinks we [older women] don't know anything and she doesn't need our support. She doesn't even talk to us nicely. I am happy to be with my mother. The conversation we have is different. I can't read or write. This is why my daughter-in-law would not follow my advice. Urgen

The influence of education in terms of how knowledge and power is perceived and acted upon in relationships is evident in these narratives. This not only created negative impacts on childbirth experiences but also led to mistrust between mother-in-law and daughter-in-law.

For Sanju, a daughter-in-law, this relationship was a distressing one.

She [mother-in-law] used to fight with me for no reason. She takes everything negatively. I did as much work as I could do. She has never been happy with me. She didn't care about my childbirth. I was restless the whole night long. She didn't come to offer any help or ask how I was going. Sanju

These experiences made it clear that we cannot sustain any relationship without mutual trust and respect. Even when there was a lack of understanding in the relationship, daughters-in-law still expected support and care from their mothers-in-law during childbirth. Not getting that support and care resulted in feeling abandoned.

The mother-in-law Lali shared her perspective and explained why she did not offer support to Sanju.

> She doesn't talk to me. I am her mother-in-law. She should respect me. Why should I go and talk to her? I heard she gave birth in the health post. She didn't call me for help, so I didn't go to her. I haven't seen her since she had this baby. If she thinks that she doesn't need me; I don't need her either. I am fine with living apart, so we don't have to fight every day. She needs to learn to respect and listen to me. Lali

Both mother-in-law and daughter-in-law had expectations of the relationship. However, the perceived lack of respect and open communication in their relationship resulted in anxiety, conflict and misunderstanding.

Sunita, a daughter-in-law shared a similar experience of her relationship with her mother-in-law.

> We don't have a good relationship. My mother-in-law is always complaining about me. We live in the same house, but we don't talk. Most of the time, she listens to other people in the village and makes unnecessary comments about me. She never asks me how I am feeling. Sunita

There has been a tendency for each party to blame one another for not establishing or sustaining a good relationship. In a conflicting relationship, the mother-in-law thought that the daughter-in-law should understand her position and take responsibility for maintaining a better relationship.

Mother-in-law Seti shared her view.

> During my childbirth, my mother-in-law did everything for me. I always shared my feelings, discomfort, and problems with her. I respected her. We looked after one another. I followed her advice all the time. Now, if I say something, she [daughter-in-law] takes it wrongly and she doesn't listen to me. It has been a year since we have talked to one another. I haven't said bad things to her, but she doesn't follow my advice. This makes me sad. Seti

These examples validate the role of mothers-in-law as oppressors exerting power over their daughters-in-law. The gap in understanding did not only influence the way in which the daughters-in-law experienced childbirth, it also impacted the perceived status of the mother-in-law to play their part in the relationship.

Chameli, a mother-in-law, expressed her concerns about lost social status.

These days Buhari [daughters-in-law] don't respect their Sasu [mother-in-law]. They do things according to their own whims and ideas. They don't ask us anything. We have been working hard our whole lives. Now it should be our time to rest. But they don't take care of us. We don't like to see Buhari not respecting their Sasu. We don't like these modern times which are rendering our existence worthless. They treat us like nobodies. It may be good for them to go to hospital to give birth, but they should respect tradition. Chameli

While a few mothers-in-law felt a loss of respect in their relationship threatened the status and power, some daughters-in-law also expressed their own difficulties. Suntali mentioned how their expectations were different.

When my husband was helping me to do household chores, my mother-in-law didn't like it. She wanted me to do everything. I didn't make any comment when she compared my work with what she did in her time. I just ignored her and started living in a separate house. Now, she has her way and I have my way – we are better this way. Suntali

Living together with your in-laws is a common feature of the joint family in Nepal. There is a social expectation that the daughter-in-law should take care of other members of the family [21]. While relationships with the mother-in-law might not work out well, having a supportive husband means a lot to these women. Although mothers-in-law have set expectations of how they would like to be treated in the relationship, some daughters-in-law were able to accept these expectations as common features in sustaining good relationships.

The relationship between daughter-in-law Rita and mother-in-law Fulmaya was sustained through the acceptance of differences.

Rita normally doesn't live with me. She came here last week; I don't know what she is doing or planning to do. I haven't asked her, and she hasn't told me. This is the difference between Sasu [mother-in-law] and Buhari [daughter-in-law]. I want her to tell me as I am her Sasu. She might be thinking differently, but how do I know? Fulmaya

Fulmaya raised a good question about communication in the relationship and how her accepted status formed expectations. Rita, the daughter-in-law, was able to understand such differences but still found it hard to find an equilibrium.

We have differences in understanding. This is problematic. My mother-in-law is different, and she has always been like that. I don't blame her though. This is the way she sees her role and I want to maintain that. Times are different, so her thinking is different to mine. I am trying my best not to disappoint her, but it isn't easy. Rita

Despite the difficulties of managing social and family expectations, there was an attempt by daughters-in-law to maintain a good relationship.

Kabita, another daughter-in-law, spoke about how she maintained expectations.

> I have been working at the school and managing household chores. It isn't easy, but I can't leave the housework undone and run off to school. As a daughter-in-law, I need to meet social expectations. In our society, a daughter-in-law can't behave like a daughter. The nature of the relationship and expectations are different. I don't want to upset my mother-in-law. I will do whatever it takes to make her happy. Kabita

These examples of a compromised relationship with acceptance of differences kept the status and power that mothers-in-law hold unthreatened. While the reciprocal relationship contributed to maintaining the status of mothers-in-law, the perceived loss of power among mothers-in-law created tensions and conflict in a relationship. Where the relationship was disrupted, the daughters-in-law felt distressed, isolated, confused and anxious about childbirth. However, negotiations in understanding were beneficial to sustaining a good relationship.

The relationship between mother-in-law and daughter-in-law is built through negotiation, trust and respect. Giddens's [24] notion of trust supports the essence of the relationship to minimise threats. For these women, trusting the knowledge and support of mothers-in-law contributed to enhancing positive childbirth experiences. So, the power that mothers-in-law hold was the outcome of good relationships.

Childbirth support: trust to knowledge and experiences

The crucial role of a support person during childbirth has been discussed previously. It has been argued that social structures and agency play a paramount role in making choices and decisions. I used this concept of structure and agency to analyse the relationships and support in childbirth.

Hodnett et al. [25] argue that continuous support from a family member is beneficial to ensuring a safe childbirth experience. For remote mountain women, support from a known and trusted person during childbirth was important. Given the different nature of relationships, when it came to childbirth, the trusted support person was their mother-in-law.

Laxmi spoke about the trust she has in her mother-in-law to support childbirth.

> My mother-in-law helped me to give birth. I trust her. She knows what to do when. I feel comfortable with her. I feel confident that nothing will go wrong when she is there. Laxmi

Respect and trust in the knowledge that mothers-in-law hold in relation to supporting the birth is significant in ensuring safety. Even when women needed to go to hospital to give birth, they wanted their mother-in-law to come with them.

Having the presence of her mother-in-law contributed to Sumi feeling safe.

> My mother-in-law helped me to give birth. If she hadn't been there, I would've had no idea about giving birth. I could've been dead. She knew everything and I felt comfortable with her. She did everything for me and my baby. It went well. Sumi

Trust in childbirth support is important to minimise possible threats. Their preference for choosing a mother-in-law to support childbirth provided a sense of safety to women.

Hira felt the absence of her mother-in-law to support childbirth.

> I feel unlucky for not having a mother-in-law. I have no one to share my difficulties or feelings with. Others who have their mother-in-law seem confident about childbirth. I don't have that confidence. Sometimes I think that my baby wouldn't have died when I gave birth last time if my mother-in-law were around. I really miss not having that support available to me. Hira

Lacking support from the mother-in-law created a sense of insecurity for women. The support of a mother-in-law was expected even when the relationship was conflictual. Sanju talked about the impact of her relationship on making choices about the place of birth.

> I wanted to give birth at home. But it was difficult without the support of my mother-in-law. She was with me when I gave birth last time. It was a great experience. But this time, my mother-in-law didn't come to support me, and I had to go to the health post. I didn't feel good about it. Sanju

The preference for having a mother-in-law supports childbirth related to trust in their knowledge and the sense of safety that women were able to experience. This helped to minimise worries and discomfort about giving birth.

Toma talked about the physical and emotional benefits of the support.

> My mother-in-law told me not to worry about giving birth. She supported me wholeheartedly. She was confident that I would be fine, and that things would go naturally. It really made me feel comfortable. Toma

This feeling of confidence that women were able to gain during childbirth was significant to determining ownership of their experiences. These women wanted their mothers-in-law to be part of their childbirth experiences.

Kabita mentioned how she followed the advice of her mother-in-law.

> When I had my first baby, I was with my mother-in-law. She knew when and how the pain started and what needed to do to comfort me. She gave me warm drinks, an oil massage and asked me to walk around. I did what she

said. I didn't have to worry about anything. It was incredible to have her supporting the whole process. Kabita

Mothers-in-law were the trusted source of childbirth knowledge and their support in facilitating the birthing process enhanced the perception of safety when giving birth for these women. As per Giddens [24], uncertainties arise from a lack of trust in information or knowledge. Women were able to develop trust in the support provided by their mothers-in-law to reduce fear of uncertainties during childbirth. The involvement of the mothers-in-law in supporting childbirth was welcomed and valued by the daughters-in-law. In this supportive relationship, the status of the mother-in-law was respected and the power they held contributed to generating shared and safe childbirth experiences.

Alternate preference: mother, aunty or sister

The first preference of women for childbirth support was the presence of their mother-in-law. When the support of the mother-in-law was not available, they wanted their mother to be part of their experience. Having mothers present to support the childbirth of their daughters is a rare option for married Nepalese women because once married, they are expected to live with their husband's family. Only those women whose mothers lived nearby had the opportunity of gaining their support during childbirth. For some women, when mothers-in-law were not available, they chose their mother as the trusted person for childbirth support.

Urgen was one of those lucky women to have her mother supporting birth.

> My mother supported all my births. I never called anyone from outside. I felt lucky to have her with me. My mother knew what can make the birth comfortable and how to manage problems. I had a great experience. Urgen

In Western societies, the uniqueness of the mother-daughter relationship involves role development, support and emotional attachment [26, 27]. In the remote mountains, this relationship is critical to supporting childbirth. Unlike the complexities resulting from the power dynamics of the mother-in-law and daughter-in-law relationship, the nature of mother-and-daughter relationships was always understanding and nurturing. Hirsch [26] noted the importance of increased emotional attachment between mother and daughter during childbirth.

Only a few women experienced the support of a mother. Dolma had the opportunity of being with her mother while giving birth.

> My mother helped me to give birth. My grandmother was also there to offer support and advice. They were experienced and skilled. They knew exactly how to handle the situation. I didn't have any problems giving birth. I felt comfortable with their support and care. Dolma

This trust in knowledge, skill and support contributed to making childbirth a safe experience. This perception of safety was lacking when similar support was not available for some women.

Toli shared her feelings of uncertainty about forthcoming childbirth.

> My mother-in-law died before I came to this house. So, my mother was with me during my first birth. She did everything for me. Being with my own mother is the best thing for me. This time, she lives far from the village and can't come to help me. I am not sure how I am going to give birth without her. Toli

The desire of women to be closer to their mother to talk about pregnancy and seek childbirth support was common.

When that desire was not met due to restrictions set by the mother-in-law, Suntali felt disappointed.

> My mother-in-law didn't let me go to visit my parents. When I got pregnant, my mother wanted me to spend time with her. I also wanted to go and stay with her. There were feelings I could only share with my mother. But my mother-in-law didn't let me go. It was very hard for me. Suntali

When the trusted person was not available for advice and support, it created worries and insecurities about childbirth outcomes.

Rita felt the absence of her mother to share experiences with.

> I felt the absence of my mother to share ups and downs with. It became intense once I got pregnant. I have no one to share my feelings or problems with. It is a different relationship and the care a mother provides to her daughter isn't comparable. I would've loved to stay with my mother to give birth if she were alive. Rita

Given the structures and expectations around married women in Nepalese society, having your mother present to support the childbirth was a special privilege which only some were able to experience. On the occasions when mother or mother-in-law were not available, women preferred experienced female relatives to support the birth.

For Tolma, it was her aunty.

> My aunty supported my births. I feel very comfortable with my aunty. She lives nearby and she knows what help is needed during birth and how to comfort the pain. She is like my own mother. I could've died while giving birth to triplets if aunty weren't there. She means everything to me. Tolma

Having someone approachable with the knowledge and experience that women trust to support the birth was consistently mentioned in these experiences. Whether it was the mother-in-law or the mother or the aunty, these characteristics were common when seeking support to give birth.

For Kiru and Lashi, the trusted person to support birth was their sisters.

> I went down to the Goth and tried to give birth by myself. The pain became more intense, and the baby wasn't coming out. I felt exhausted. Then, I asked my daughter to call my sister, as she doesn't live far away. She came and helped me. She has been the one I call for help when needed. Kiru
>
> I had pain for three days. Ani [my sister] was there with me the whole time. The baby came in the evening of the third day. Ani did everything for me. I didn't have any problems. I didn't have to worry about anything. Lashi

The preference for and choice of the support person was linked with the family and childbirth circumstances. Some women tried giving birth without a support person and some sought help when needed. Their preferences were based on the knowledge, accessibility, experiences, skill in providing support, trust and comforting nature of the relationship. On all occasions, they preferred women to provide childbirth support. Although the supporting person had control of the birth, the issue of power did not occur because the help provided contributed to gaining a safe and comfortable birthing experience.

Heath [28] argues that reciprocity and mutual trust in the relationship enable the negotiation of power through shared understanding. This was evident in the stories shared by women as their relationships evolved around negotiating the nature and extent of support they received during the childbirth. When women trust other women for their knowledge and skills to support the birth, the power they held to control the birthing process was accepted making childbirth a shared collective experience.

A supportive husband: what does it entail?

Gender in patriarchy is a traditionally embedded social structure which values male power over female. This notion of gender and power makes the relationship between men and women more complex to understand. In Nepalese society, a relationship generally starts with a formally arranged marriage. A married relationship is considered a social contract with set expectations which define the role of a husband and wife. Undoubtedly, the husband takes control and exerts power over the wife making her voiceless and oppressed. The way this relationship is perceived and practiced in society impacts how women experience pregnancy and childbirth. The relationship between husband and wife in terms of making childbirth decisions has been widely contested. Since childbirth has been considered a women's matter, men's involvement is not socially encouraged and admired in South Asia. The role of a husband in childbirth has not yet been a commonly discussed agenda. This became evident in this research as many husbands did not want to talk about childbirth.

In Nepal, because of the pollution beliefs, the husband is not allowed to touch the wife or go inside the birthing place. Because of limited involvement in these matters, they lack knowledge about childbirth and problems that could happen while giving birth. In this context, their presence during birth is about being around and being part of decisions in case an emergency arises [29]. Despite men's reluctance to engage in childbirth, an increasing desire of women for the involvement of their husbands during childbirth has been evident [30, 31].

Even though men were excluded from the birthing space, having their husband around was important for women to feel emotionally safe and the lack of that presence caused distress and loneliness.

Lashi shared her feelings.

> I felt so lonely. I wished he [husband] was with me. I felt weak and there was no one to take the sick baby to the hospital. If he were here, he could've done that, and I wouldn't have had to worry. Although men don't understand a lot of things about birth and babies, it is still good for a wife to live with her husband. They [men] aren't weak [emotionally and physically] like us. I feel helpless and insecure without him. Lashi

Given that many births take place within the home environment, the role of husband was not about facilitating or comforting the birthing process but was critical to managing problems if medical help was required. So, the concept of a "supportive husband" was a commonly expected feature in the relationship.

Rita explained the role a "supportive husband" plays in childbirth.

> He [husband] is a good person. He worries about me all the time and regrets not being around to support me. Before he left for overseas, he asked other people to help me if anything went wrong during birth. The feeling of being with him is different and nothing replaces that absence. He calls every day and tries to comfort me. I miss him a lot but can't ask him to come back. He needs to earn money before coming home. I just need to hope that nothing goes wrong. Rita

In a patriarchal social structure, financial responsibility sits with men. So, the trend of male migration to urban areas and overseas for financial purposes has been a common phenomenon in Nepal. Husbands come home once a year to visit their wife if they are working in urban areas. If they are working in another country, the visit occurs every three years or longer. Usually, the pregnancy occurs during those visits and women are left behind by their husband to go through it all. Given the interest in staying together, women accepted that temporary migration is a required role for a husband and appreciated the emotional and financial support provided for their comfort.

Understanding each other better is the key to any relationship. It is normal for women to feel vulnerable while going through a new experience such as childbirth. In addition to support and care, Sarita pointed to the importance of mutual understanding.

> I am so happy with my husband. He understands and supports me. Unlike other men in society, his caring attitude is unique. He knows about childbirth

and what needs to be done to keep mother and baby healthy. He can decide what to do and when to do it. He looks after me very well. He thinks both men and women are equal. I feel lucky to have him as my husband. Sarita

Changing attitudes towards gender play a significant role in the husband-wife relationship. A husband who treats his wife with respect and provides the care she needs is the best outcome for a woman. This is only possible through social change around the gender norms constructed for men and women. This shift towards gender equality opens ample opportunities to change expectations by giving more power and respect to women in a patriarchal society. A caring relationship should not be a matter of luck for women and attempts to create a culture of treating women as equal must be made. Without question, women are keen to experience a relationship that is caring, respectful and supportive.

Sarita's husband, Ramesh explained why he has acted differently to others in society.

I have seen many newborn deaths in the village. I have also seen a mother die after giving birth. I was anxious about Sarita currently. I was worried about birth outcomes. That is why we decided from the start to have regular check-ups and to give birth at the hospital. I don't know many men in the village think about their wife or children. We need to change this male mindset. I am happy that both Sarita and the baby are healthy. We are a happy family. Ramesh

The knowledge that a husband held and the positive nature of the relationship were critical in deciding about the birthplace and the care required. This decision seemed appropriate to minimising the anticipated risks of adverse birth outcomes. This is consistent with other studies reporting the involvement of husbands in providing childbirth support to improve positive birth outcomes [32, 33] and making decisions about seeking medical care to reduce the risk for mothers and babies [30].

Even though decisions to take appropriate action when births did not progress normally were made by husbands, women considered that part of a supportive relationship and no comments were made around power differences. The role of a husband in making decisions and seeking timely medical care to lower the risks of negative birth outcomes was a lifesaving support for many women.

Rima explained how her husband took charge of making decisions about care.

He [husband] is very good. I would be dead if he hadn't brought me to the hospital last time. He managed to fly me out to the city, and I was able to give birth. I survived. His support has always been great. This time, he decided to come to the city hospital early to make sure that I could give birth safely. Other husbands don't care about their wife or support them this way. I am grateful to my husband. Rima

The ability to make decisions about care is based on knowledge and experience. When a husband can make appropriate and timely decisions to seek medical care, it helps promote the survival of mothers and babies. This indicates that educating husbands about childbirth and associated risks could help reduce the high incidence of childbirth-related mortality and morbidity.

Rabin, Rima's husband, spoke about how the knowledge he gained through experience, education and his religious orientation enabled him to play a supportive role.

> I think the role of the husband is crucial during pregnancy and childbirth. Rima left her family and came to spend the rest of her life with me. I should take responsibility for looking after her well. I should be the one to be part of her grief and happiness. In the Bible, they wrote that when your wife leaves her family to marry, then it is your responsibility to make her happy with love and care. I follow the Bible and offer my love and care to Rima. My contact with educated circles and conversations about relationships with them made me realise the need to respect women. I am doing my best to make Rima happy and comfortable. I think this is what all men should do for their wives – show them respect, love, and care. Rabin

The husband as care provider is not a socially accepted role in Nepal. Rabin is an example of the positive and supportive role a husband can play for their wife. His realisation about treating women with respect and invitation to other men do the same opens opportunities for transformation and confirms that childbirth is not only a women's agenda. The combined approach of education and religion has been successful in creating positive childbirth supports [34]. In childbirth, knowledge and understanding of a husband helped women to recover from traumatic experiences [35].

Structural gender inequalities manifest in husband-and-wife relationships resulting in conflict, sexual abuse and violence. The physical and emotional abuse of a husband is not often spoken about in patriarchal society due to the expectations that men have the right to control women. Most women accept their status within the social structure and follow expectations to perform the role of a "good wife and a daughter-in-law." Fertility decisions and choice did not reside with women. Being ready to have sex with the husband whenever asked was a socially demanded and desired expectation. In a married relationship, women were not able to question or deny that sexual expectation.

Although women in these societies do not openly talk about sex, abuse or violence in married relationships, Pema mentioned the torture she received from her first husband.

> I had a very hard time. I had to work all day and go through the physical and emotional torture of my husband during the night. When I gave birth to my daughter, there was no one to help me. My husband – he was drunk. He was shouting at me to bring more food and more drinks. I gave birth in such difficult conditions. Pema

Marriage in a patriarchal system sides with men and often blames women for causing problems or violence in a relationship. In married relationships, women do not only become the victim of abuse by their husbands, but they are also further victimised by society for not following stereotypical social expectations. Breaking a marriage and leaving the relationship is not commonly accepted in society. As men's control over women is accepted, women tend to stay in marriages even if the relationship becomes toxic. Pema was brave enough to decide to leave her first husband and marry Chiring. This is an exceptional example, and the relationship with her second husband was supportive. The understanding and care she received from this husband made a difference to her childbirth experiences.

> Now, I am so happy with Chiring. He loves me. It feels like heaven compared to the experience with my former husband. Although we are not rich, we share the pain, comfort, and happiness together. I still work hard but I sleep soundly during the night. He pays attention to me. I love this life. I am happy now. I am not worried about childbirth if he is around. Pema

The mutual understanding and support of their husbands provided a sense of security for these women. However, it was not easy for those husbands who wanted to play a supportive role in the circumstances when resources were not available. Chiring, Pema's husband talked about the complexities.

> I know she [wife] is weak. I also know that she needs to eat enough vegetables, do light work, take care of pregnancy, and have enough rest. I can't provide that to her as we don't have food available in the village. We can't grow or buy vegetables here. We have children to look after and she is going to give birth soon. I am wondering how to manage the work when she needs to rest after giving birth. It isn't easy for us here, but I am with her to share pain and happiness together. Chiring

Zadoroznyj [36] relates material circumstances to birthing choices and argues that social class has a strong influence on the childbirth experiences of women. Although the context of women in remote mountain areas is socially complex, the influence of structural determinants in childbirth remains critical. Nevertheless, the safety that women were able to experience through the care and support of their husband is important to consider. The influence of the husband in making decisions about medical care to manage risk appeared to be the significant action in promoting maternal and newborn survival. This finding opens the possibility of involving men in playing a more active role in childbirth.

These experiences confirmed that both social structures and human agency had strong influences on childbirth. Within the patriarchal social structure, most relationships silenced women about their choices and expectations. While managing risks and getting help to support childbirth, these relationships were beneficial to women. Women spoke strongly about the comfort and sense of security gained through the support of their mother-in-law, husband and other female relatives during childbirth confirming the benefits of structural relationships. At the same time, women were also the victims of structural oppression and chronic control. This created a complex paradox for understanding the influence of power in these socially structured relationships and roles. Given the social circumstances, the dynamics of structural relationships and the influences of power were gradually changing. In a positive relationship, the power that people hold to support childbirth was accepted by women. This acceptance of support contributed to the collective ownership of experiences.

There was an interplay of a form of power in married relationships which restricted women in making decisions about their childbirth. The legitimate power that a husband holds within the familial structure created a form of coercion making women oppressed within the relationship. However, mutual understanding, respect and trust enabled the sustaining of supportive relationships in both familial and social structures. Giddens [37] highlighted structures can constrain or enable certain forms of behaviour. The influence of chronic patriarchy in defining the role of "powerful men" and "submissive women" was apparent in the husband-and-wife relationship. Although women accepted their subordinate status within society, they desired to be treated with respect inside and outside the household. The nature of power that individuals portray at familial or societal levels was linked with this knowledge, defined roles and experiences. Trust was the core factor in making relationships supportive, caring, respectful and understanding to women.

Outside home: who to trust and why?

A complex array of relationships had strong influences on childbirth where people holding a higher status in social or formal structures had authority to exercise power. In local terms, women referred to those people who held a higher social status as "the big people" [Thula Manche]. These people did not only have social status, but they were also able to gain respect and trust. Their role in childbirth was not directly related but they were influential in offering advice or contributing to decisions. The respect given to the people with social status in the village was linked to the knowledge they held.

For example, a school teacher held a respected social status in the village, and he was the main source of advice even for health-related matters. The school teacher, who villagers called "the Head Sir," spoke about this trust in local knowledge.

> If they [village people] get sick, they don't go anywhere without consulting me or their Lama [local religious leader]. If I give them medicine to treat their problems, they think it will work better because I am the teacher [the head sir]. They trust me. They also trust the medicine given by their Lama. If a local health worker gives them the same medicine, they don't think that it is effective to treat their illness. This is how villagers see medical care. School teacher

This illustrates that trust in knowledge is based on the source of knowledge rather than the knowledge itself. In cases, where local religious leaders and school teachers are influential in decision making about care, it is more complicated for women to trust healthcare providers in regard to care and support during childbirth.

As is the case with household relationships, trust in specific people outside the home developed through a shared understanding. A local Indigenous leader was the other respected person who people trusted for both traditional and medical knowledge.

The Indigenous leader talked about how trust in knowledge and care is constructed and practised in the village.

> When there are health problems, people look to the Lama [religious faith leader] and other local traditional healers. They are more comfortable with them than with health workers. I haven't got any training in providing health care, but I've been helping them with basic problems. I usually buy medicines and keep them at home. In the village, when people are sick, they come to me. They don't go to the health post. The villagers don't like health workers complaining about their hygiene. So, I've been like a doctor in this village. I know childbirth is different and I can't manage problems in giving birth. A few women died while giving birth in the village. I tried my best, but I couldn't save their lives. Even if I tell them to go to the hospital, they won't go. It is my Dharma [duty] to help them and I've been doing that for the last 20 years. Local Indigenous leader

There was a two-way dynamic of respect which contributed to establishing trust in relationships. The understanding of the context of the village by stakeholders has been significant in gaining the respect and trust needed to offer advice and care. In contrast, the health workers were unable to gain similar trust and respect because of the blame they directed towards the villagers for their living conditions. Given the context in which they lived, the trend towards blaming the community for their health was problematic.

In relation to childbirth, trust in knowledge did not only sit with the people holding highly respected positions, but there were also other community-based care providers who women tended to reach out to for advice and support. FCHVs and TBAs were roles which gained trust and respect from women. A FCHV who was also trained as a TBA spoke about the preferences of women in the village.

> Women feel comfortable to share their problems with us [FCHV and TBA]. They don't like talking about their problems with family members, so they prefer us. They feel shy going to a health post for a check-up, normally there are male health workers. They don't like sharing their problems with men. Three women in the village gave birth recently and I helped one of them. Family members don't want to take women to the health post. Instead, they call us at home when help is needed. I do Sudheni work as well [Traditional Birth Attendant], so they trust me. There are other Sudheni as well in the village who can help. Local FCHV

The preference of family members to choose a TBA during childbirth is a common practice in Nepal [38, 39]. The FCHVs are trained by the health system to provide advice and refer the women to health institutions for childbirth. Although the government invests in training TBAs to provide safer care to women, those who were doing Sudheni work in the village were not trained but their birth support knowledge was developed through experience.

Traditional Faith Healers were another group of care provider in the village. They were mostly men locally known as Dhami [Shaman]. There was a strong belief and trust in the healing performed by these Shamans to treat health-related and quite often childbirth problems. The respect towards Shamans was associated with their traditional knowledge and healing practices.

A local faith healer spoke about the preference for traditional healing practices.

> Most of the time, villagers call me to perform the ritual when someone is sick in the family. They will call when women go through childbirth problems as well and I perform the same ritual to make them feel better. They trust me and the healing I perform, so I need to go and help them when needed. In case I am not around, they will look for another Dhami [Shaman] to treat the condition. They don't like to go to hospital. Even if I tell them to go and see the doctor, they don't want to do that. I will continue to support them with my Dhami knowledge. Traditional faith healer

The preference for traditional healing was linked with a respect for and trust in lay knowledge. During the conversation, Sunita's mother-in-law spoke about how she valued traditional healing over medical care.

> Two weeks ago, we were all working, I was bleeding. It continued. On the fifth day it became serious and I was unconscious. They took me to a pharmacy at around midnight and then to the district hospital. I had a few injections and transfusions. I returned home the next day. These injections made me weaker and I didn't feel better. So, I started going to the Dhami [Traditional Faith Healer]. He said this is all happening because of the "Nepale Hawa" [Nepali Air]. I am gradually starting to feel better. Going to the hospital was a waste. They should have just called the Dhami to wake me up. Seti

This experience confirmed the trust in traditional healing by women in the village. The reason for lacking trust in medical care was linked with the effectiveness of care to treat the condition. In this example, medical care failed to heal a woman which led to the preference for a traditional faith healer who was able to provide comfort and a positive experience.

The influence of stakeholders was not limited to offering advice or support or care to manage health problems. They had a strong influence on making decisions about health services in the community. However, the local politician indicated that addressing the healthcare needs of the community is only possible if services and resources are available in the village.

The villagers are saying to me that they can never find a doctor [health worker] at the health post. They told me that the health post rarely opens and doesn't have any medicine. Yesterday the father of a sick child went to several health posts trying to find medicines, but he couldn't get any. Then, he bought medicines from a pharmacy (which was about 6 hours away). Sadly, the baby died before he reached home with the medicine. Most of our children are sick now but there is no help. This is a serious problem in the village. I want to make sure that services are available, but health workers don't come to the village. I am aware of the problems and trying to reassure villagers. The only option they have is consulting the Lama and local care providers who are in the village. Local politician

Political responsibility is important in tackling the social determinants impacting the health and well-being of populations. It is reasonable to argue that the health system plays the major role in addressing the factors leading to poor health outcomes in resource-limited settings. Local politicians held a powerful status but could not sustain trust and respect because they were unable to take appropriate action to increase access to services and resources in the community. Given the circumstances of people living in complex social conditions, this is a human rights issue which needs prioritising by the government.

Different perspectives and influences shared here reveal trust as the core factor in respecting the knowledge and status that people held in the community. These people were trusted by the community to provide positive support, effective care and appropriate advice. The influence these people had on the community contributed to developing a shared understanding and positive experiences for women.

Left uninformed: the professional control of birth

Childbirth stories women shared in this research explored the differences between the concept of safety and risk in childbirth. The differences in the construction of risk knowledge in medical and cultural paradigms impacted the childbirth experiences of women where healthcare providers-controlled childbirth marginalising women during the birthing process. Most women gave birth at home but those who needed to seek medical help for various reasons shared negative experiences.

The obstinate attitude of some health service providers left women confused, hence there were unknowns about their condition. Sarita shared her experience.

I went to the hospital for regular prenatal check-ups. The services they provided to us were not good. They only see women on Wednesdays. Usually, many women line up for check-ups. They [health workers] don't give enough time or attention to each woman. They didn't tell me anything – nothing about pregnancy or the condition of the baby. I was curious to know what they found from the check-ups, but they never told me. They wouldn't even answer my questions. I didn't feel that I was listened to or valued. It was meaningless to go there. I was mostly frustrated. Sarita

Making a day-long walk to the hospital for a prenatal check-up yet returning home without the knowledge of how their pregnancy is progressing added to the disbelief in medical care to enhance childbirth safety for these women.

Toli shared a similar experience about her visit to the hospital for a prenatal check-up.

> I went to the hospital once for my prenatal check-up. They didn't check me properly. There were many women and I had to wait a while for my turn to come. She [midwife] palpated my abdomen. She asked me something, but I didn't understand. I didn't follow what she was asking, and she became irritated. She was angry at me. I told her I didn't get what she asked but she walked off without saying anything. She didn't tell me anything about the baby or pregnancy and whether I needed to come back again. I shouldn't have gone for a check-up. It was a waste of time and energy. After that experience, I haven't been back to the hospital. I don't see any point in going there. Toli

The dominant power held by healthcare providers left women uninformed about their own condition. As a result, women lacked respect and trust in the medical knowledge, institutional care and care providers.

Manu spoke about her experience of a prenatal visit.

> I had only one check-up. I went to the hospital on a Friday. They asked me to wait until Wednesday for a check-up. Instead of walking back to the village the next day, I decided to wait until Wednesday. Finally, the long-awaited check-up was done. But the sister didn't tell me anything. I wanted to know how the pregnancy was going. The sister said, oh you have a big belly. I had no clue what that meant as she didn't explain anything. She gave me a piece of card and called another woman for a check-up. There was no explanation or conversation. I had to leave home for a week for that check-up and got no information or advice about the childbirth. Manu

Healthcare providers treated these women in a mechanical way with no respect to their status or condition. The way that women were treated did not only decrease trust in medical care, but further increased the sense of uncertainty and insecurities about childbirth. In some instances, women felt threatened by the healthcare providers.

Jitu mentioned how she was threatened for not making prenatal visits to the healthcare centre.

> They [health workers] said that I must go for prenatal check-ups. If I didn't go for check-ups, they would send the police to my house. The other woman who went to the health post for a check-up brought that message to me. So, I went to the health post once and had the check-up. I didn't get anything out of it. They asked me to come back, but I didn't like going there again. I didn't see any reason why they wanted me to come there regularly. Jitu

The coercive power used by the healthcare providers indicates the mechanistic control of women's experiences which women refused to be part of because it threatened the perception of safety. Furthermore, the differences in how childbirth was viewed and controlled in institutional settings made women very uncomfortable.

Rima shared how she felt being in that controlled environment.

> After several hours' travel from my district, I found myself in a completely different place. It was an unknown and unusual place to me. The hospital was different, people were different and the way they talked was also different. I felt uncomfortable talking to them. I was in pain and discomfort. They tried different injections. I didn't know why I needed those injections. The only thing that came to my mind was that they were trying to save my life. I didn't question anything, and no one explained to me what was happening. It was all different to me. I wanted to give birth on my own. But on the third day, they decided to do the operation and took me to the theatre. It was so scary. Everything was happening like a machine. Rima

Kitzinger [40] argues that the use of technology and medicalisation of birth in an institutional setting tends to dehumanise women's birthing experiences. These mountain women felt excluded from part of their own experience when procedures were employed without a conversation or discussion with them to explain what was happening to their body. Professionals mostly made decisions based on knowledge of the medical risks during childbirth, while women were forced to follow instructions for the survival of themselves and their babies [41]. Consequently, women felt like they were with a stranger in a highly oppressive, voiceless and neglected institutional environment.

Suntali was a trained midwife and attended the local birthing centre to give birth. She found the care unsafe and felt neglected by the healthcare providers.

> In the birthing centre, initially they told me that I would be fine. Later, they said something different. At one stage they told me the cord was tied around the baby's neck. At another stage, they told me that I had a contracted pelvis. As labour progressed, they told me that I wouldn't be able to give birth normally. It was confusing what was happening and what they were saying, I was disappointed. There was no reassurance or comforting conversations. They even blamed me for not going to the city and getting a video x-ray done. How was that possible? A health worker [auxiliary health worker] came and started giving oxytocins. I noticed that he gave me 10 units of oxytocins initially and didn't maintain the actual drops. He knew I am a midwife but didn't explain anything. I felt that I was going to die in that place. So, I asked my husband to take me to the hospital and he did. The staff in the birthing centre were hopeless. I had a very bad experience. I can't expect them to do the right thing for women. It was their negligence. There is no way that I can trust them. I wonder what would happen to other women who go there. It would be even worse. Suntali

The oppressive attitude and inappropriate treatment of healthcare providers created mistrust in institutional care. The control and negligence shown by professionals towards this qualified midwife, call into question the competencies of care providers to manage childbirth and the role institutions play in providing safe experiences for women.

The professional power that healthcare providers held to control the childbirth experiences of women was confirmed while I interviewed the doctor. The language he used portrayed the structural marginalisation of community people and the medical intention to control the childbirth experiences of women.

> The socio-economic condition of the people in the district is not good. They are poor and uneducated. The status of women is more complex in the mountains. In peasant farming families, they need somebody to do the work. Mostly these workers are women. So, they want their sons to get married and bring in women to work for the family. This means a girl must get married and join the husband as a working member of the family. Then, education and knowledge are another factor. Unless people are educated and aware of the risks associated with pregnancy and childbirth, we can't help them. They need to know the reasons for coming to the hospital for antenatal check-ups and to give birth. They don't know anything about why they need to take certain injections, prenatal vitamins, and other special nutrients. Unless they have some knowledge of medical care and a willingness to come to the hospital to give birth, we can't save their lives. There are multifactorial influences when it comes to childbirth for women in the mountains. My message to all women is they must come to hospital or seek support from health workers to give birth. That is the only way we save the lives of mothers and babies. Medical doctor

This was a power-laden comment with a one-way strategy for the survival of mothers and babies in the mountains. Asking women to come to the hospital to give birth contradicts the interests of many women who preferred staying home.

Unlike the controlling tone of the medical doctor, the local midwife was sympathetic towards the circumstances of women and explained the reasons why some women started coming to the hospital.

> Women started to come to the hospital only after they knew that they would get money [cash incentives]. There were only five women who came here last year. This year, we already had more than 30 women coming to give birth. This trend is increasing. Some gave birth at home and came to the hospital due to the bleeding or retained placenta. Although we've been telling them to come to the hospital for check-ups and to give birth, it hasn't been happening. Only women who live nearby are coming to get the cash incentive. This had made a positive impact on safe childbirth but still there are many women who haven't been able to come to the hospital. Local midwife

The cash incentives programme that the Government of Nepal introduced had some impact on increasing rates of institutional childbirth. Women receive the cash payment while attending health institutions to give birth. Paradoxically, going to the health institution is not what women in this study wanted for their childbirth. The incentive programme created an indirect pressure on the family to bring women to healthcare facilities to give birth. An interesting aspect of this scheme was that service providers received a higher amount of cash incentive when the birth was attended in an institution compared to a home birth. Women who had home births were not eligible for any incentives. This programme influenced women's choices and decisions about childbirth for the benefit of health workers more than the women themselves. This prompted healthcare providers to blame women for not choosing healthcare facilities to give birth.

> The women in the village don't know anything. They don't know the safe way of giving birth. They are 16th-century people, still giving birth in the Goth. Though several organizations are working here to change their lifestyle, it has had no impact. Women still do the same thing. I have been telling them to come to the health post and reminded them many times about the risks of giving birth in the Goth. They don't come. They like their old-fashioned tradition. Local health worker

A victim-blaming attitude from healthcare providers emerged consistently and impacted the provision of care to women. There was a clear power difference in the relationship, and the provider-recipient relationship in this context was dysfunctional and disappointing for some women. The powerful influence of healthcare professionals within institutional settings distorted women's experiences. This power and control by health professionals rendered women helpless, voiceless and powerless in their own experiences of childbirth.

Young [42] points to power differences existing in society and how they influence the way people make decisions. Women trusted local and traditional care providers to seek advice and support for their childbirth-related problems. There was two-way respect and understanding in these local relationships. In these instances, their influence was positive and trusted by women. In contrast, when health workers exerted their power over women, they failed to gain their respect and trust. This paradoxical power relationship significantly impacted the women, as they felt oppression within the institutional environment and their trust in traditional care providers stayed stronger. The notion of collective action became possible through positive and supportive relationships.

Trust and respect were paramount for a reciprocity of understanding [43], where the function of trust contributed to reduce fear and uncertainties around childbirth. Women received support and advice from a trusted person to make decisions about the care required to manage childbirth-related problems. A lack of trust in medical care and healthcare providers has emerged from the negative experiences of women in an institutional environment. The victim-blaming attitude, coercive power and marginalisation of women during the birthing process were the main factors leading to the mistrust of medical knowledge. As Lupton [44] pointed out, childbirth was controlled by expert knowledge and the legitimacy of the healthcare providers, resulting in an oppressor-oppressed dynamic.

Conclusion

Childbirth is a powerful experience for women. Birthing experiences of women in the remote mountains of Nepal is influenced by both social structures and agencies. More importantly, various forms of relationships existed in the society and were influential in relation to childbirth. These influences impacted women to enhance or diminish their sense of safety during childbirth. Similarly, there were social norms, roles, expectations, tradition and knowledge within socially constructed structures to interact in these relationships. The interplay between the structures and agency indicated that the status of women and their relationships within and outside the household were crucial to childbirth. This demonstrated that despite the submissive status of the women in the society, women-to-women relationships were critical to childbirth support.

A multiplicity of relationships that mountain women related to had paradoxical power interactions which led to complexities, contradictions and negotiations in constructing collective birthing experiences. Various forms of social relations were influenced by ideological and material conditions of gender, knowledge, status quo and social position. Furthermore, the socio-political process shaped the healthcare system and policies to operate against the choices and preferences of women, making services inaccessible in cultural, physical and social terms. The perception of safety during childbirth in the institutional environment was diminished as women felt threatened by the practices and the environment itself. Consequently, women were reluctant to seek medical help and a reliance on traditional knowledge and support remained valued. This again highlighted the significance of a collaborative model of care to meet social, cultural and medical needs to promote maternal and newborn survival in this socially complex and culturally rich community.

References

1   Davis-Floyd, R., *The technocratic, humanistic, and holistic paradigms of childbirth.* International Journal of Gynaecology and Obstetrics, 2001. **75**(1): p. S5–S23.
2   Oakley, A., *Childbirth practice should take women's wishes into account.* British Medical Journal, 1996. **313**(7071): p. 1557.
3   Weingarten, K., *The discourses of intimacy: Adding a social constructionist and feminist view.* Family Process, 1991. **30**(3): p. 285–305.
4   Rothman, B.K., *Women, providers, and control.* Journal of Obstetric, Gynecologic, and Neonatal Nursing, 1996. **25**(3): p. 253–256.
5   Cockburn, C., *On the machinery of dominance: Women, men, and technical know-how.* Women's Studies Quarterly, 2009. **37**(1/2): p. 269–273.
6   Croson, R. and U. Gneezy, *Gender differences in preferences.* Journal of Economic Literature, 2009. **47**(2): p. 448–474.
7   Scott, J.W., *Gender: A useful category of historical analysis.* The American Historical Review, 1986. **91**(5): p. 1053–1075.
8   Stern, S.J., *The secret history of gender: Women, men, and power in late colonial Mexico.* 1997: University of North Carolina Press, Chapel Hill.
9   Martin, E., *The woman in the body: A cultural analysis of reproduction Milton Keynes.* 1989: Open University Press, Berkshire.

10   Regmi, K., R. Smart, and J. Kottler, *Understanding gender and power dynamics within the family: A qualitative study of Nepali women's experience.* Australian and New Zealand Journal of Family Therapy, 2010. **31**(2): p. 191–201.

11   Watkins, J.C., *Spirited women: Gender, religion, and cultural identity in the Nepal Himalaya.* 1996: Columbia University Press, New York.

12   Thompson, C., *Women, fertility and the worship of gods in a Hindu village.* Women's Religious Experience. 1983: Barnes and Noble, New York.

13   Panter-Brick, C., *Motherhood and subsistence work: The Tamang of rural Nepal.* Human Ecology, 1989. **17**(2): p. 205–228.

14   Gautam, S., A. Banskota, and R. Manchanda, Where there are no men: Women in the Maoist insurgency in Nepal, in K. Visweswaran, *Perspectives on modern South Asia: A reader in culture, history, and representation.* 2011: Blackwell Publishing, Oxford.

15   Kandiyoti, D., *Bargaining with Patriarchy'.* Gender and Society, 1988. **2**(3): p. 274–290.

16   Lein, L., *Male participation in home life: Impact of social supports and breadwinner responsibility on the allocation of tasks.* Family Coordinator, 1979. **28**(4): p. 489–495.

17   Treas, J. and S. Drobnič, *Dividing the domestic: Men, women, and household work in cross-national perspective.* 2010: Stanford University Press, Palo Alto.

18   Zuo, J. and S. Tang, *Breadwinner status and gender ideologies of men and women regarding family roles.* Sociological Perspectives, 2000. **43**(1): p. 29–43.

19   Rai, N., *Constitutional development of gender equality issue in Nepal.* 2010: Kathmandu School of Law, Kathmandu.

20   Freire, P., *Education for critical consciousness.* 1973: Bloomsbury Publishing, London.

21   Simkhada, B., M.A. Porter, and E.R. Van Teijlingen, *The role of mothers-in-law in antenatal care decision-making in Nepal: A qualitative study.* BMC Pregnancy and Childbirth, 2010. **10**(1): p. 34.

22   Cameron, M.M., *On the edge of the auspicious: Gender and caste in Nepal.* 1998: University of Illinois Press, Champaign.

23   Manandhar, M., *Ethnographic perspectives on obstetric health issues in Nepal: A literature review.* 2000: Options, London.

24   Giddens, A., *Risk, trust, reflexivity.* Reflexive Modernization, 1994: Stanford University Press, Palo Alto.

25   Hodnett, E.D., et al., *Continuous support for women during childbirth.* Cochrane Database of Systematic Reviews, 2013. (7).

26   Hirsch, M., *The mother/daughter plot: Narrative, psychoanalysis, feminism.* 1989: Indiana University Press, Bloomington.

27   Martell, L.K., *The mother-daughter relationship during daughter's first pregnancy: The transition experience.* Holistic Nursing Practice, 1990. **4**(3): p. 47–55.

28   Heath, R.G., *Rethinking community collaboration through a dialogic lens: Creativity, democracy, and diversity in community organizing.* Management Communication Quarterly, 2007. **21**(2): p. 145–171.

29   Brunson, J., *Son preference in the context of fertility decline: Limits to new constructions of gender and kinship in Nepal.* Studies in Family Planning, 2010. **41**(2): p. 89–98.

30   Sapkota, S., et al., *In the Nepalese context, can a husband's attendance during childbirth help his wife feel more in control of labour?* BMC Pregnancy and Childbirth, 2012. **12**(1): p. 49.

31   Sapkota, S., T. Kobayashi, and M. Takase, *Impact on perceived postnatal support, maternal anxiety and symptoms of depression in new mothers in Nepal when their husbands provide continuous support during labour.* Midwifery, 2013. **29**(11): p. 1264–1271.

32   Kakaire, O., D.K. Kaye, and M.O. Osinde, *Male involvement in birth prepared-ness and complication readiness for emergency obstetric referrals in rural Uganda.* Reproductive Health, 2011. **8**(1): p. 12.

33   Sawyer, A., et al., *Women's experiences of pregnancy, childbirth, and the postna-tal period in the Gambia: A qualitative study.* British Journal of Health Psychology, 2011. **16**(3): p. 528–541.

34   Stambach, A., *Education, religion, and anthropology in Africa.* Annual Review of Anthropology, 2010. **39**: p. 361–379.

35   Khan, T.M., et al., *Role of the husband's knowledge and behaviour in postnatal depression: A case study of an immigrant Pakistani woman.* Mental Health in Family Medicine, 2009. **6**(4): p. 195.

36   Zadoroznyj, M., *Social class, social selves and social control in childbirth.* Sociology of Health and Illness, 1999. **21**(3): p. 267–289.

37   Giddens, A., *Risk and responsibility.* 1999: Blackwell Publishing, Hoboken.

38   Osrin, D., et al., *Cross sectional, community based study of care of newborn infants in Nepal.* British Medical Journal, 2002. **325**(7372): p. 1063.

39   Rhee, V., et al., *Maternal and birth attendant hand washing and neonatal mortality in southern Nepal.* Archives of Paediatrics and Adolescent Medicine, 2008. **162**(7): p. 603–608.

40   Kitzinger, S., *Some cultural perspectives of birth.* British Journal of Midwifery, 2000. **8**(12): p. 746–750.

41   Torres, J.M. and R.G. De Vries, *Birthing ethics: What mothers, families, childbirth educators, nurses, and physicians should know about the ethics of childbirth.* The Journal of Perinatal Education, 2009. **18**(1): p. 12.

42   Young, I.M., *Justice and the politics of difference.* 2011: Princeton University Press, Princeton.

43   Luhmann, N., *Trust and power.* 2018: Wiley and Sons, Hoboken.

44   Lupton, D., *Risk and sociocultural theory: New directions and perspectives.* 1999: Cambridge University Press, Cambridge.

6 A complex array of factors
Too far and too hard

Introduction

Where did you carry that load from Didi? I asked the woman walking beside me with a heavy load on her back. There were two children walking alongside her with small carry-on loads.

"Gamghadi [District Headquarter]. The government supplied rice from there yesterday and we went to collect it," she responded.

"It is a long way to walk with the loads," I commented.

"Yes, it is but we don't have options. We have no food in the village. We usually go to China to buy things we need for the year. Going to the markets in China is closer for us," she added.

"Did you say China?" I asked.

"Yes, we can get to China in about five hours. Going to Gamghadi takes double time and we need to plan a two-day trip. We need to go too far just to get everyday things. Our life is too hard sister. This might surprise you." She looked at my face and paused.

Compared to those living in Nepal's urban areas, people living in the remote mountain areas have particularly poor social, economic and health status with chronic food insecurity [1] and higher fertility, morbidity and mortality rates [2]. Although there is much documentation concerning issues of access to services in rural and remote villages in Nepal [2–5] what remains unanswered is the interplay between social, cultural, political and structural factors and the birth outcomes. The influence of the broader social factors on maternal, newborn and perinatal survival is a critical issue in Nepal's remote villages [6].

Social determinants of health influence the ability for women to reach maternal, newborn and child health services in many countries [7, 8]. According to the literature, most services offered in institutional settings are either not accessible to women or inequitably distributed [9, 10]. Women living in remote settings are unable to access services because of the associated cost of travel, time limitations and their everyday household responsibilities [11, 12]. These factors have been consistent barriers to accessing services for women living in remote Nepal [4, 13–15].

The influence and interrelationship of cultures, traditions, social values and different forms of power are critical to childbirth experiences of women. It is evident that women internalise the importance of cultural safety and generational transfer of knowledge about childbirth. It is also clear that despite the risk to their survival during childbirth, women preferred giving birth in the community. Women trust traditional knowledge and local support for their determination to stay home to give birth. I will provide further accounts of women to explain why they preferred to give birth at home as opposed to giving birth in a healthcare setting. Hearing from women about their experiences of being in the healthcare environment raised concerns around their perception of safety. While examining the preferences of women about the place to give birth, a complex array of factors emerged which favoured community setting and questioned the attempt of the government to institutionalise women for giving birth.

Going to the hospital: place of institutional birth

Women spoke about their preference to give birth in the local community as opposed to in the healthcare or institutional settings to minimise risks. Some women raised a serious question of how the institutionalised approach to childbirth fits within the socio-cultural context of women where childbirth is a collective social experience.

Juna shared her concerns about going to hospital to give birth.

> We do not like to go to the hospital to give birth. We will go to the hospital when we cannot give birth at home. The pain is the same wherever we go. If we can give birth ourselves at home, why do we need to go to hospital? I do not see any point in going to hospital. Staying home is better for us. We have our people around and we can do things as we like. We can get hot foods and put on the fire to feel warm. We do not get these choices in the hospital. This is far better than walking many hours. Why do they want us to go to hospital just to give birth? Juna

Having ownership of the birthplace and birthing process is an important part of childbirth experiences to these women. The benefits articulated by Juna confirm that women have more choices and supports to make childbirth comfortable when they give birth within their home environment. Giving birth in the village further signified the cultural importance by allowing women to gain collective ownership of experiences.

Sumi reinforced the benefits of giving birth at home.

> When I gave birth at home, I was able to ask for the things (food, drinks, oil massage) I wanted to have. I was able to do the things I wanted, and my mother-in-law asked me to do. My mother-in-law was with me to help give birth. She never made a loud voice or said bad things. I had to go to hospital to give birth this time, they never asked me if I wanted anything to make birth better. They only came to check unnecessarily and said the heartbeat of the baby is a bit slow. I was in higher pain and they asked me to stop yelling.

I had to be quiet and follow them. I had no choice to do anything. They did not let the mother-in-law massage my back. They gave saline and a few injections which I think was not required. I would have been better off not going to the hospital. Sumi

The institutional control of birth restricted the choices that women wanted for their comfort and safety. Not allowing traditional practice and support of family members was concerning for Sumi. This demonstrated a clear difference between home births and hospital births in terms of women's experiences. Although Laxmi had problems during the birth and was taken to hospital to manage the problems, she did not feel safe there.

I preferred staying at home to give birth. Home is better and more comfortable. I did not have to worry about anything while giving birth at home. My mother-in-law brought me here for a check-up. I had a little bleeding and they said bleeding is a big risk and admitted me. Nothing wrong happened apart from that little bleeding. I was confident to give birth normally at home. But they said it is a high risk to the mother and baby. I must stay there following their advice. It was not my choice. I still think that I can give birth by myself at home. Laxmi

The medical notion of risks limited women's ability to experience birth according to their wishes and forced them to follow the practice of institutional birth. Culturally, women were determined to experience normal home births. Following the traditional knowledge and seeking support of their mother-in-law to give birth remained the preferred choice for these women.

Some of the women who had gone to hospital for a number of reasons developed a negative impression about the way the care was provided to them.

A husband from the village shared his experience of taking his wife to district hospital.

I took my wife to the hospital because we were in doubt whether everything was going well. They did not do anything. The baby was moving around. She could feel the movement. They [nurses] said; the baby was dead inside and did nothing. I brought her back to the village. She gave birth and the baby was alive. You can see – still very healthy [pointing the child]. It made me think that these nurses knew nothing. They made us anxious and stressed about the situation. Hearing that your baby is dead – it was not a joke. Then we decided not to go to hospital anymore. We are better ourselves in the village. Prakash

In the remote mountains, travelling to the healthcare facility or district hospital was neither a simple nor cost-efficient option due to the time, distance and household commitments. It was disappointing when women tried to seek medical help and ended up with more distressing experiences. In this example, ineffective care and information provided by the midwives and healthcare professionals led to the serious concerns about the trusting of the medical system.

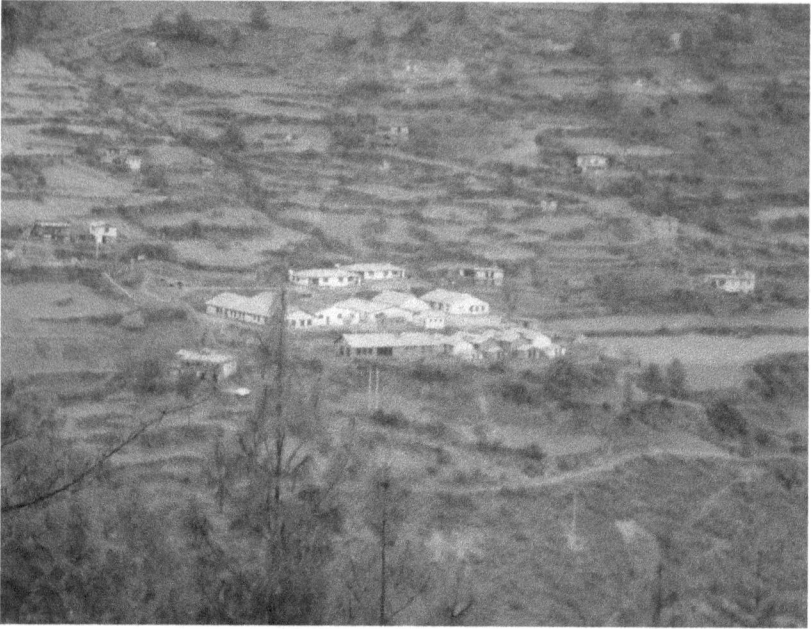

Figure 6.1 The only hospital in the district that women are expected to come to give birth
Source: Picture taken by the author

As the childbirth was considered a socially and culturally significant experience, the villagers were not in favour of the medical notion of risks. The authority of healthcare providers and the language used to describe the risks, or the problems involved during childbirth were not welcoming and comfortable to women who gave birth in medical institutions.

Rabin explained how the pregnancy was considered risky.

> The doctor said, "Rima's [his wife] is short and young, so she is at risk of giving birth normally. She is in the high-risk category and needs an operation. She won't be able to give birth in the district hospital and you need to take her to the city." So, I took her to the city and the baby was born via operation [Caesarean Section]. Rabin

The form of power and control that women and family members experienced in this research was consistent with Kitzinger's [16] critique of medicalised birth which puts women in the risk category of having complications and medically monitors their labour and birth. Although the possibility of having a normal birth in those circumstances has been well documented [17, 18], there was no opportunity given to discuss the options of having normal birth, as the decision about caesarean section was made based on risk categorisation. Davis Floyd's [19] critique of medicalised birth in which women's bodies are considered as a machine was evident for remote mountain women experiencing institutional births. Women's experiences of medical control of birth in institutional settings led to the increased trust to continue traditional birthing practice.

Poor remote women: structural oppression and social disadvantages

Women and the family in the remote mountains challenged the medical construction of risk and expressed their concern about safety while giving birth in the institutional setting. Given the social circumstances, it was clear that going to hospital was not the appropriate solution to address the issue of maternal and newborn survival. They introduced their status as poor, uneducated, disadvantaged and remote mountain women. A significant influence of geographic remoteness, poverty and ongoing food insecurity was revealed in their experiences.

Hira described her life in the village.

> We are poor remote women [Durgamka Garib Mahila]. We are not educated. We have not seen the city. We do not know about life outside this village. We have not seen motors. Our task is to get married, get pregnant, give birth, raise children, and get enough food to feed the family. We are stressed everyday about the food. We cannot think of anything else unless we get food for the family. Women normally do not get enough food to eat. Hira

It was difficult for women to stay healthy and strong to give birth when there has been a consistent lack of food for everyday life. The villagers were not able to produce enough food for the whole year due to the high-altitude topography and extreme cold weather. The food supply from the urban area via helicopter has been tried but was not a reliable option. Local suppliers often use mules [locally called Khachad] to transport food and other essential supplies from district headquarter to remote villages.

Generally, women walk to the administrative headquarters of the district for several hours to fetch rice supplied by the government which was enough for three months of the year. In a culture where women also eat last in the family, they tend to not get a decent amount of food at any point including during pregnancy.

This issue was raised by Sonam as well.

> We are living in very remote areas with not enough food to eat. We are very poor and cannot afford to buy more food. We do not know anything as we are not educated. We do not know why our children died and are still dying. The only thing we know is that they die because they were sick and did not get any treatment. The doctor does not come here because it is too far and too hard for them to live in the village. Sonam

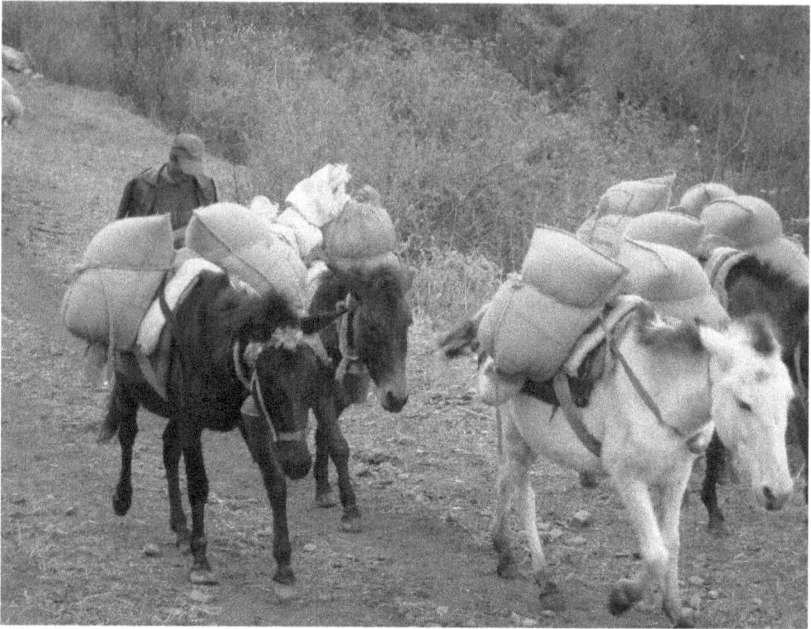

Figure 6.2 Local transport option to carry food and other supplies to the village
Source: Picture taken by the author

Dolma highlights the issue of not having enough food to eat, which in turn required them to work hard and not rest during pregnancy.

> We live far away from the city. We do not have enough food to eat. We need to work hard to feed the family and we do not have time to take a rest. We live in poverty and the government does not care about us. They want us to go to Gamghadi [District Hospital] when we are sick. We have nothing in the village. Dolma

For most women with the consistent pressure of maintaining household chores and feeding the family, it was not feasible for them to attend services which are far away, and one suggested that medical staff could perhaps come to them instead. Even if services were free, taking women away from their daily routines on long trips to and from the hospital added further risk to their physical and emotional well-being.

The social circumstances had an impact on women and girls of the mountains. The complexities around childbirth, survival of mothers and babies did not only relate to the place of birth or the support during childbirth. The broader social factors created the condition to make women more vulnerable. The socio-cultural practice of marrying young was one of the factors that increased vulnerability.

A local politician commented about the social practice of early marriage of girls.

In the village, people think that it is better to send the girls off to their husband's home, as it releases the burden for the parents. They usually marry their daughter very early. This helps to manage the cost of food, as there will be less people in the house. It also reduces the social burden, as there is an expectation that the young daughters should not be staying with parents. If they [parents] do not arrange the marriage of their daughters, other people start to criticise for not being able to find a boy to marry. It is a social expectation for girls to leave their parental house before the age of 15, in most cases before they had their first period [menstruation]. How can we expect change in this context? [He laughed]. Local politician

The local journalist recognised the power of social practice, which overrides the law for early marriage. He commented about the trend of early marriage practice among girls and its impact on women.

In Karnali, a girl becomes older without experiencing their pubertal age. They are usually married by age of 12. The trend of early marriage is common, and it is affecting their reproductive health. There is a direct link of early age marriage of girls and poor birth outcomes of women. Their girlhood turns quickly to womanhood – married young and pregnant. It impacts the health of both mother and baby. We have been advocating to end the early age marriage practice, but it is not changing. The early marriage is the main problem here if we are talking about women's health. There is a legal age of marriage but enforcing the law does not really do anything to social practice. The change should come socially first. There is another correlation I found that the early marriage is increasing because of the food scarcity. They want to send their daughter off as early as possible. This is a serious issue needing attention by all sectors. Journalist

The social and structural issues emerged in this research need a serious consideration to address effectively. Although the legal age of marriage for girls in Nepal is 18 years, it does not have any effect on social practice. This is tragic when a young girl experiences the sexual burden and becomes pregnant without her body being physically mature for it. This issue of structural oppression and social disadvantage that women experience could be resolved with a sustained strategy for long-term investments across all sectors.

The medical doctor further commented about the risks associated with the young age of marriage.

The situation of childbirth in the district is like a complex wave in the ocean. Because of the ignorance and various socioeconomic constraints, girls are getting married at a young age, like the age of 10, 12, 13 or 15 years. They become pregnant at a very young age. Teenage pregnancy itself is high-risk.

> There are lots of problems associated with teenage pregnancy. Unless the girls are married at an appropriate age when they are physically and mentally mature, the risk of maternal and newborn deaths continues. Medical doctor

This could be a reasonable argument that there are risks associated with teenage pregnancies, but the structural constraints that women experienced must be addressed appropriately to ensure the survival and safety around childbirth.

The deep-rooted structural oppression on the ground of social characteristics made women think that expecting positive change in their life is unrealistic and impossible. Lashi spoke about it categorising herself as a poor lower caste woman.

> I am a poor lower caste woman. Women from lower caste are treated differently everywhere. We are poor and marginalised in all senses. Even the health workers treat us badly. Improvement is not possible in our life. We will be living in the same way for many years. No one speaks in the favour of a lower caste woman. Rich people are always rich and poor people are always poor. This is the way it is. I do not expect any change in the way we are living. Lashi

Other community members also raised the issue of power and discrimination against the ethnic and geographic background. The Lama community is an Indigenous group in Nepal. Chiring mentioned the inequalities.

> There is an unequal treatment to Indigenous people. Although the government is saying that the Indigenous people should be the priority of any interventions or programs, other caste people dominate Indigenous people. Brahman, Chhetri and Thakuri [higher caste groups] people are in administrative positions and they hold the power in the district. They make decisions in their favour. Indigenous people have limited access to resources and services. The system does not respect the needs of Indigenous people. Yesterday, I saw a big poster with a message that everyone is equal, but I do not see that in practice. So, it is better for our women to stay in the village while giving birth. We can help each other, and we can share whatever we have locally. Even the workers in the hospital treat us differently. Mostly the workers there are from Brahman and Chettri background. They say that Lama people are dirty and smell bad. We are better ourselves. Chiring

In remote mountains, the access to services and resources was influenced by the social background of the populations where the power sat with the higher caste people. On the one hand, Lama people were discriminated against, and on the other hand, there was an impression that the services were not designed for them. Jitu thinks that these services are for higher class people.

> Only those people who are living around the hospital can go to hospital to give birth. Going to the hospital is not possible for us. You [people who often

use hospital services] must be either rich or live nearby to use hospital services. The hospital is too far. Leaving work and children behind is too hard
for us. Jitu

The issue of rural women's physical access to services has been a challenge in
reducing maternal and newborn mortality in Nepal [20, 21]. Women shared additional social and structural issues which were limiting their access to services. The
issue of poverty in terms of maternal and newborn health was further highlighted
by Pema.

> The mothers and babies are dying in the village. We think this is happening
> because we are poor. We do not have money to go to the hospital on time and
> wait for the baby to be born. We cannot do that. The doctor [health worker]
> comes to the village and tells you to do different things. They say you should
> do this and that. They do not give us anything. All people [health workers]
> come to say their things, ask their questions, and leave. This does not help to
> change our situation. Pema

This was a valid critique about the inability of health workers to understand the
socio-cultural conditions of the people. Their assumptions around the association
of poverty with adverse birth outcomes was consistent with other evidence [22, 23].
   Sonam had to walk for three days to access services needed to manage the risk
of dying. Sonam acknowledged the need for medical help but blamed her own
ignorance and remoteness for the difficulties in seeking services.

> We are living in very remote areas. We do not know anything. Our children
> are dying because of not getting treatment and not having a doctor in the vil-
> lage. We tried using Lama and Dhami [Traditional Faith Healers] but it did
> not help. I had a difficult time giving birth. I had to walk for three days with
> pain and discomfort to get to the district hospital. Being in the remote moun-
> tain, this is what we must go through. This is too hard. Sonam

When a few women went through the experience of loss of their newborn babies,
they realised the importance of medical care to prevent these deaths. Toli thought
her triplets could have been saved if she were in a city hospital with specialised
better-quality services.

> If I were in the city, my babies would have survived. I heard this type of
> babies can survive in city hospitals. Nothing is available in the village. No
> one thinks about us. Thinking about the better care being made available in
> the village can only be a dream for us. It is not possible to go to the city to
> give birth. Toli

While exploring the social, cultural, physical and financial barriers to services
in the remote mountains, the criticality of poverty in terms of accessing food

and basic resources appeared to be a significant determinant to healthy outcomes of childbirth for mother and baby. Labonte's [24] socio-environmental approach with the involvement of other sectors to enhance health opens the possibility to address the complexities related to the socio-cultural circumstances of the women in the mountains.

Marmot [25] described the social inequity in maternal health in which he highlighted the social, economic and political factors influencing the higher burden of deaths in developing countries. The WHO and UNICEF [26] emphasises the influence of political, social, economic, technological and environmental factors in reducing mortality and promoting maternal and newborn health. Low SES and the long distance to the hospital have been found to be the key barriers for women going to the hospital to give birth in rural areas of Nepal [27]. The remote mountain women raised the issues of geographic distance to the hospital, social distance between them and healthcare workers and their socio-economic conditions as the barriers to accessing services. Thus, the participants' expectations of making services available to them at the village was important to take into the account at both policy and practice levels.

What are they saying? Policy, practice and reality

The influences of structural, social and political determinants are critical to ensure childbirth safety of women [28–31]. Maternal health has been a major focus of new public health initiatives with the emphasis on addressing structural factors to ensure equity in utilisation of health services [32, 33].

Overcoming geographic inequity in the utilisation of services has been a critical barrier in promoting maternal and newborn health in many developing countries [34, 35]. However, remote mountain women raised the serious issue of accessing health services given the social and structural dimensions of their everyday life. The geographic context not only restricted women from accessing care they needed but also limited their ability to manage basic resources for everyday survival including food. Consequently, a tension existed for women when they were informed about the need for hospital care and good nutrition without making those services and resources available to access.

Tolma shared her experiences.

> They [health care providers] said that we should eat better food. We should take enough rest. We should go for regular check-ups in the hospital. But this does not apply to us. They do not understand our situation and they only tell us to do things. How can we do regular checks, as we do not even have a nurse in the village? We are struggling to feed family and children. How can we eat better food? We are working 24 hours to run the house. We cannot rest when we have so many things to handle in our life. Tolma

Telling women what needs to be done without enabling the environment for that to happen disrupts dialogue and raises a social justice issue. This issue of health workers not understanding the context faced in remote villages was raised by Rima, with a hope that services could perhaps be provided in the village.

> The health workers do not understand that we like our tradition, and we are happy to stay in our village to give birth. We are comfortable here. It would be better if they [health workers] do not ask women to go that far when things go wrong. It would help to have a doctor or nurse in the village if they are serious about us. Why do they just come to tell us what needs to be done and leave the village? This is not helping us. Rima

Toli commented about the lack of health services and support in the village.

> We have a health post [health care centre] only in the name in the village. It is all useless. It never opens and health workers never come to work from the health post. We need to go to a medical shop [pharmacy] in the district headquarter to seek advice and buy medicines. We heard that the government supplies medicines in the health post, but we cannot get them here. Toli

The physical disadvantage of accessing basic health care due to the unavailability of services being provided in the village highlights the criticality of addressing structural and system barriers to improve maternal and newborn health outcomes. It seems impossible and unfair for these women to walk through difficult terrains of multiple mountains while they are heavily pregnant or when they are going through severe labour pain to access services available in the hospital.

Getting medical help has not been an easy solution to these women living in the remote mountains. Chiring explained the difficulties he encountered attempting to manage the problems his wife was experiencing during childbirth.

> We have no health workers in the village. This is the big problem. I told the Madam [MCH worker] the other day that she should come to the village and check my wife. Instead, she asked me to bring her to the hospital. I cannot take her to the hospital to give birth. It is too far for us. We will stay home and wait for the baby to be born. Going to hospital is too hard for us. Who will look after these children at home? The health workers supposed to stay here to provide services never do so. This is quite frustrating. Chiring

In this scenario, the health workers were reluctant to come to the village and the villagers were unable to access services located in the hospital because of social, cultural, financial and physical reasons. Despite an ongoing attempt to improve coverage of community-based maternal and newborn care services in Nepal [21], these communities were experiencing a consistent lack of services.

Sonam shared her recent experience.

> The nearest health centre we have is in Pulu [adjoining village which is also three hours' walking distance], but there are no doctors [health workers]. I went there the other day but could not find anyone. There was no stretcher.

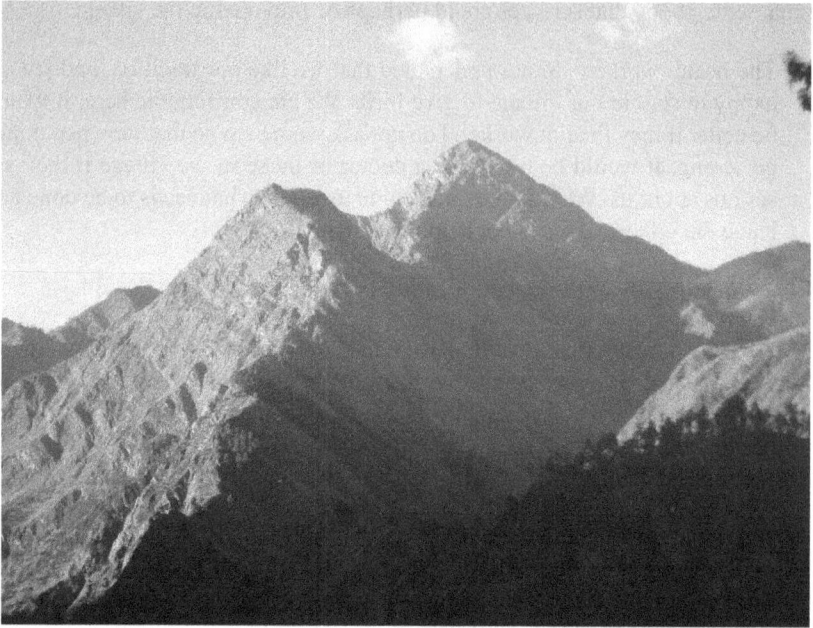

Figure 6.3 Landscape of mountains that women require to walk to access services
Source: Picture taken by the author

> It took me two days walking slowly to reach hospital. It was costly to rent
> a room and stay in the Gamghadi [district headquarters]. We were worried
> about the children at home and we also missed the cropping season. The hos-
> pital is not an option for us. Sonam

In a situation when women needed to go to the hospital, the transfer was difficult
due to the lack of resources and long walking hours. Although several attempts
had been made by different organisations in collaboration with the government
to create a maternal and child health fund for emergency transport [36, 37], no
evidence of that initiative was found in the remote mountains. Petchesky [38]
highlights that critical feminist practice needs to focus on women's rights and
social circumstances. These women were informed that their traditional childbirth practice was risky, but they were not given access to safe maternity care
to give birth. This reflects the contradiction and the complexity of balancing the
childbirth tradition and managing associated risk childbirth. Although the feminist critical approach affirms that women's health must be treated as an end, not
merely as the means towards other social goals, many dimensions of the lives
demonstrated that there were no such options available to women to ensure their
right to survival during childbirth.

Nevertheless, this research offered some emancipating possibilities to promote childbirth safety. Labonte [24] argues that the medical approach is important but insufficient, and this research acknowledged the possible risks during childbirth and appreciated the importance of medical help to manage these risks. From the community side, women and their family members saw the possibility of collaboration between culture and medicine for promoting safety. The concept of shared understanding and shared responsibility seemed very important not only between men and women but at all levels of relationships. However, the related power issues created a gap which is possible to address through a dialogical approach for collective actions.

Who takes responsibility? Political context and potential for change

The social and structural constraints, including the limitations of the healthcare system to provide access to services to the women in the remote mountains has been an ongoing challenge for maternal and newborn survival. A situation of no one claiming the responsibility of maternal and newborn health with a tendency to blame each other for the consistent lack of services emerged.

A local Indigenous leader shared his view.

> We are aware that there must be services available to women to use during childbirth. The services must go hand in hand with the awareness raising programmes at the community, so women are aware of the care needed. However, both services are not available in the village. There is a plan to establish a birthing centre, but it is also not in an appropriate location. This village is the centre for all surrounding villages, but the political leaders decided to open the birthing centre in another village. Our women will not be able to go there. Few women will be able to use that birthing centre. This is not a good effort of the government or these leaders. The local politicians do the things in their favour and ignore the community. When the leaders do not take things seriously and make right decisions for the broader community, we cannot do anything. Local Indigenous leader

Political power has become an issue in which the community has no choices or involvement to make decisions about the services. In Nepal, the actions are taken according to the interest of the political party rather than the priorities of the policy of the government. Thus, priorities also change, once the government changes. So, the local Indigenous leader blamed the political manipulation of decision-making which constrained the women to access childbirth services. Although promoting maternal and newborn survival has been a political priority in Nepal [39], it has not been translated into practice yet. This indicates that the politicians are not taking responsibility for women's access to childbirth services.

A local politician made the following comments about the government.

In mountain districts, there is the consistent lack of health services. Mostly people have no education and lack of appropriate advice. Still, there are strong cultural beliefs and traditional practices where people trust more in Traditional Faith Healers. The health of mothers and children has remained a serious problem in the district and especially in this village. In urban areas, we do take care of women offering good food, rest, and special attention during pregnancy. We do not have such options in the village. Most of the women in this village are suffering from childbirth related problems. I asked for services to be co-located in the village, but the government made the decision to make a birthing centre in another village. This is the worst scenario of political power. Local politician

The issues of political power in terms of ensuring access to services in the community has been important to consider by the health service system. The centralised power dynamics led to inappropriate interventions without considering the needs of the community. The local politician did not claim it was his responsibility to facilitate the process of improving access to services. A blame for their trust to the traditional healing system posed against women with the need to educate them about the appropriate care raises a critical question.

Rabin spoke about the role of education for better childbirth experiences for women.

Without education, they [men] cannot understand the pain and discomfort that women go through while giving birth. They [men] do not know how childbirth takes place and what type of care needed for women. Educated men can understand this better and take care of their wife. Education teaches them to value women. But you know sister, in our village [he laughs], it doesn't even matter for them losing their babies. They take it easily as though nothing had happened. Rabin

The acknowledgement of the role of education and its contribution to promoting childbirth safety was significant to minimise the possible risks associated with childbirth. The responsibility of men to take care of women for safe childbirth experience has been a solution to address the higher mortality. However, the blame made against the community for not being able to do so needs consideration while developing appropriate interventions.

Ramesh believed that education could contribute to influence positive change.

This is a remote area, but education could play an important role for social change. The social, economic, and educational status of people living in this area is very poor, which makes everything hard. Personally, I have not been able to do what I want. I want to see the positive change happening. But I have not been able to talk about changing the social practice. No one will listen to me. So, I think education has the power to influence change. Ramesh

Ramesh was optimistic about achieving changes through education. Educating the community members including both men and women can be the means of changing social practice, which could help to increase the chances of maternal and newborn survival by making childbirth a safe and satisfying experience.

A local journalist emphasised the importance of education and raised awareness for women in the mountains.

> The poor status of women's health in the district is related to education. The mountain region is far behind in literacy levels. There is a direct link between education and awareness of people. Educated people could possibly be aware of health care needs to prompt appropriate actions. Most of the women are illiterate. They do not send girls to school. Most of the mountain communities have the same problems. Journalist

Freire's conscientisation process emphasises the need for education through the involvement of community people [40–42], which is liberating and empowering rather than subtly imposing conformity to another set of values and practices. Freire's [40] approach to education focuses more on enabling the social transformation of oppressed groups of people through dialogical cultural actions. In his approach, individuals can construct their own set of values and knowledge and so, there is room for the people to decide which knowledge they want to construct for their benefit rather than it being imposed by external knowledge. Considering the culture and tradition in the mountains, Freire's [40] approach could offer some possibilities for protecting lay knowledge and sustaining traditional practices while gaining new knowledge of risk.

A local high school teacher described the need for different forms of education.

> The situation of having high maternal and newborn deaths in the mountains is due to the lack of awareness among the people. When I first came here, they [villagers] were more interested in sending their sons to become Lama [Chumba] than sending them to school. They believed that their sons would be able to live a happy life doing Gyan [ritual performance]. That practice is still common here. They do not believe in the modern education system. They think it has negative impacts on society, as some educated youth started doing the bad things. It is more about creating social awareness than core education. High school teacher

Creating social awareness has been an important concept to influence change. In the community where faith-based education had more value as opposed to formal education, it is important to bring both aspects of education together for negotiation around the change of social practice and tradition of childbirth.

While others saw the role of education to create positive change, Rabin thought that the responsibilities of addressing childbirth-related issues must sit with the healthcare system.

The health system should be responsible to mobilise health care resources in the mountain villages. They need to make sure that women can receive required care. They should be aware of the social conditions of women and make resources available locally to manage childbirth related problems. Childbirth is the most complicated issue in the mountains, and this must be a priority issue. It is important to keep in mind that many women and babies are dying. The health system should take accountability to these deaths. There must be programs and services in the village to prevent deaths. Rabin

The important perspective raised here confirmed that rather than blaming each other, there is a need for shared responsibility to make services and resources available to women locally. Shor and Freire [42] demonstrate the effectiveness of dialogue in action to liberating people and transforming society. Their concept of dialogue offers an opportunity to bring service providers, villagers, politicians and other social leaders for shared understanding and responsibility to childbirth.

Young [43] proposes the mediation process to address the differences in views that different people hold in the society. This process could be helpful to develop reciprocal understanding and shared responsibility of addressing the determinants crucial to childbirth in the remote mountains. Heath's [44] concept of collaborative dialogue offers further opportunity to negotiate power relationships through innovative and creative approaches. Apart from the issues of access to health services and education, there are other critical issues related to everyday survival which need to be brought to the attention of politicians, stakeholders, service providers and policymakers. The government was blamed for not addressing the factors contributing to the health and childbirth experiences of women in the mountains.

A local journalist spoke about this issue.

Mugu district was the lowest ranking in the human development index with only 34 years of life expectancy. There is an ongoing issue of food scarcity. It means that people living in this district simply do not have access to basic things. Unless the government provides access to food, shelter, and other basic services to the people, we cannot expect their health to be in good condition. Regarding the situation of the health of mother and baby, it is important to meet their basic needs first. In the current scenario, the government has not been able to do anything. The government should be accountable to address the basic rights of the people for fulfilling their basic needs of survival and ensuring their access to basic health services, resources, and opportunities. Journalist

It is important to note that the consideration of health as a human right does not only highlight the serious issue for the government to consider but also raises the critical issue of social drawbacks. This is an urgent call for the government to fulfil the basic rights of people to improve health outcomes.

A medical doctor, who represented the health system, mentioned the policy initiatives that the government had made to address the economic issues for increasing access to services.

Mugu is one of the unfortunate districts of Nepal with no connection to road networks. The transportation within the district is also very hard. However, the government has a policy of giving incentives to those women coming to the hospital or birthing centre to give birth. We give 1500 rupees (about $20 USD) to the women who come to hospital to give birth. This incentive covers the cost of carrying women in a stretcher to the hospital, which requires four to five people in the mountain district. Recently, the government put forward the policy of giving incentives to those pregnant women, who completed their fourth ANC [Antenatal Clinic] visit. I believe that this policy will increase the prenatal check-ups rate so we can manage risky pregnancies on time to take necessary actions. Medical doctor

The expectation of the medical doctor is justified in the light of the effectiveness of maternity incentive schemes in increasing utilisation of maternity services which is reported elsewhere in Nepal [45–47]. However, giving incentives to motivate women to use the services which they do not see as culturally appropriate may not be a solution to the problem in the mountains. Maternal and newborn health is a public health priority in the current healthcare system; however, women in low resource settings are still a long way behind in getting access to PHC [48]. Continuing to blame women and village people only perpetuates the problem and does not alleviate the problem of unsafe childbirth. Nevertheless, there were also emancipating possibilities shared by women and the community could be used for the development of context specific policies and strategies.

A female member of parliament nominated from the mountain region questioned the practicality of the incentive scheme and the free maternity service policy of the government.

The government has announced free childbirth services in the health post. There is also an incentive programme for childbirth service users. But this does not mean anything for people living in these remote villages. This is not practical as the services are too far from the villages. The government needs to spend more money on awareness and education programs, building more health posts, increasing numbers of midwives, improving quality of services in the hospital, and ensuring availability of health workers in the villages. A female member of parliament

Socio-cultural conditions and geographic constraints were not the only issues related to accessing services, the journalist said that the government is trying to escape from their responsibility by blaming people.

If the government takes responsibility for the citizens, remoteness is not a major problem for this country. If the government is committed, it is not hard to connect this district with the road. There are many possibilities. People [government and others] are blaming remoteness for not having better health status, this is not a fair comment. They are taking this as an excuse to ignore the issue. This is not the people's [community] fault to live in mountains. This is the negligence of the government to provide resources and services to the people. We cannot blame the place or the community. It is really an unjustified blame that the government is making to the people of the mountains. Journalist

The tendency of the government to blame people and avoid responsibility is not uncommon in Nepal. The responsibility of the government was linked to their perceived failure to consider social, structural and political factors which were critical to promote birth outcomes in the remote mountains in Nepal. There were consistent shortages of food, several hours' walk required to access basic health care, the ongoing unavailability of health workers and the burden of the cost associated with travel to access the services which were all considered as major barriers to maternal and newborn health [49]. The continued absence of health workers and lack of quality services were also raised. No consensus among service providers, politicians, other stakeholders and community was found; rather there was a tendency of blaming each other where no one was ready to claim the responsibility. In this counter blame scenario, there was no evidence of shared understanding, responsibility and accountability. Sadly, women developed an attitude of self-resignation and accepted the circumstances they were in the mountains for the problems to occur. So, it is deemed critical to establish a process for shared responsibility and collective actions to address the corresponding issues.

Ramesh, a local man again highlighted the responsibility of the government.

I think the issues related to safe birth are also related to the state management system. This is not only a local issue; the state [government] should take responsibility and give women a respected status. They should provide special places and opportunities for women. Ramesh

The call for creating opportunities for women through proper state management systems is an undeniable request that the government should take into consideration. Further complexities in relation to promoting childbirth safety where there was a contradiction in claiming responsibility were apparent in these arguments. Interestingly, none of the participants holding political and authoritative power talked about claiming the responsibility for addressing the structural issues of the mountains instead, they passed on blame. More importantly, they were developing an attitude of domination and oppression towards the community. Their views were likely to be heard by others because they have access to the arenas where they can promulgate their views, where community views were not likely to be heard in the same places.

I argue that the survival of mother and babies should be everyone's responsibility. There has been an ongoing debate about who is responsible for the health of the populations. The focus of medicine is on risk factors with the view that health is an individual's responsibility [50]. The medical concept of responsibility for health was evident in this research, in which the blame was put against the community for poor birth outcomes. Historically, even public health has focused on averting the risk factors rather than identifying the origin of the risk [51], a comprehensive PHC approach could be effective to address the ranges of factors impacting the health of mother and babies in the mountains.

Health is seen as being beyond personal and government responsibility and the 1997 Jakarta Declaration on Health Promotion into the 21st Century placed a high priority on promoting social responsibility for health [52]. Most public health initiatives are moving forward with the consensus that health is everyone's responsibility in which there is a role for the individual, family, community, and national and international governments. There is therefore a need for negotiation to develop a sense of collective responsibility for addressing the range of socio-cultural and structural determinants rather than throwing responsibility back to another level. This understanding and collective effort could contribute to ensuring women's right to health and survival during childbirth [6].

The right to health is expressed in the International Bill of Human Rights as, "the right to the highest attainable standard of physical and mental health" [53]. This right imposes a duty upon states and nations to promote and protect the health of individuals and the community and ensure quality of care. Maternal and newborn survival is also one of the human rights issues in the global public health initiative [54]. However, the right to maternal and newborn survival in the mountains was affected by many factors which the government was not managing effectively. It raises serious human right concerns about the availability of basic resources and services in the remote mountains.

Conclusion

Women's childbirth experiences are impacted by wide ranges of cultural, social, structural and political determinants which are beyond the capacity of the medical model to address while aiming to prevent the associated risks for improving maternal and newborn survival in remote communities. Women's everyday life circumstances play a critical role in childbirth and are not yet taken into the consideration while making decisions by policymakers, service providers or practitioners. The effectiveness of existing actions taken by the government to address the issues experienced by women and the community has been questionable. Given the circumstances of women, it is impossible to utilise services available in a distant location when they experience childbirth problems. This situation left women without access to basic services and resources to stay healthy during pregnancy, childbirth and postnatal period in the remote communities.

As the healthcare system continues to struggle to address the challenges that confront remote communities, broader social issues impacting childbirth outcomes must be addressed with appropriate actions. Thus, a call has been made to consider the impacts of broader determinants in everyday life of women while developing policies and strategies to enable culturally responsive, safe and appropriate services to women. Ensuring access to services, information and resources locally could help to address the causes leading to higher morbidities and mortalities associated with childbirth in remote settings.

References

1   Gentle, P. and T.N. Maraseni, *Climate change, poverty and livelihoods: Adaptation practices by rural mountain communities in Nepal.* Environmental Science and Policy, 2012. **21**: p. 24–34.

2   Khanal, V., et al., *Factors associated with small size at birth in Nepal: Further analysis of Nepal Demographic and Health Survey 2011.* BMC Pregnancy and Childbirth, 2014. **14**(1): p. 32.

3   Bennett, L., D.R. Dahal, and P. Govindasamy, *Caste, ethnic, and regional identity in Nepal: Further analysis of the 2006 Nepal Demographic and Health Survey.* 2008: Ministry of Health and Population, Government of Nepal, Kathmandu.

4   Regmi, K., R. Smart, and J. Kottler, *Understanding gender and power dynamics within the family: A qualitative study of Nepali women's experience.* Australian and New Zealand Journal of Family Therapy, 2010. **31**(2): p. 191–201.

5   Pandey, J.P., *Maternal and child health in Nepal: The effects of caste, ethnicity, and regional identity: Further analysis of the 2011 Nepal demographic and health survey.* 2013: Ministry of Health and Population, Kathmandu.

6   Kaphle, S., H. Hancock, and L.A. Newman, *Childbirth traditions and cultural perceptions of safety in Nepal: Critical spaces to ensure the survival of mothers and newborns in remote mountain villages.* Midwifery, 2013. **29**(10): p. 1173–1181.

7   Akanbi, M.A., et al., *Socio-economic factors influencing the utilization of maternal health care services in Amuwo-Odofin local government area of Lagos state, Nigeria.* International Journal of Humanities, Arts, Medicine and Sciences, 2015. **3**(3): p. 1–10.

8   Barros, A.J., et al., *Equity in maternal, newborn, and child health interventions in Countdown to 2015: A retrospective review of survey data from 54 countries.* The Lancet, 2012. **379**(9822): p. 1225–1233.

9   Aziz, A., F.A. Khan, and G. Wood, *Who is excluded and how? An analysis of community spaces for maternal and child health in Pakistan.* Health Research Policy and Systems, 2015. **13**(1): p. S56.

10   Victora, C.G., et al., *How changes in coverage affect equity in maternal and child health interventions in 35 Countdown to 2015 countries: An analysis of national surveys.* The Lancet, 2012. **380**(9848): p. 1149–1156.

11   Hanson, C., et al., *Maternal mortality and distance to facility-based obstetric care in rural southern Tanzania: A secondary analysis of cross-sectional census data in 226 000 households.* The Lancet Global Health, 2015. **3**(7): p. e387–e395.

12   Houweling, T.A., et al., *Reaching the poor with health interventions: Programme-incidence analysis of seven randomised trials of women's groups to reduce newborn mortality in Asia and Africa.* Journal of Epidemiology Community Health, 2016. **70**(1): p. 31–41.

13   Abu-Ghanem, S., et al., *Lack of prenatal care in a traditional community: Trends and perinatal outcomes.* Archives of Gynaecology and Obstetrics, 2012. **285**(5): p. 1237–1242.

14   Hodge, A., et al., *Utilisation of health services and geography: Deconstructing regional differences in barriers to facility-based delivery in Nepal.* Maternal and Child Health Journal, 2015. **19**(3): p. 566–577.

15   Simkhada, B., et al., *Why do costs act as a barrier in maternity care for some, but not all women? A qualitative study in rural Nepal.* International Journal of Social Economics, 2014.

16   Kitzinger, S., *Some cultural perspectives of birth.* British Journal of Midwifery, 2000. **8**(12): p. 746–750.

17 Carroll, C.S., Sr., et al., *Vaginal birth after caesarean section versus elective repeat cesarean delivery: Weight-based outcomes.* American Journal of Obstetrics and Gynaecology, 2003. **188**(6): p. 1516–1522.

18 Chen, L., et al., *Influence of acculturation on risk for gestational diabetes among Asian women.* Prevalence of Chronic Diseases, 2019. **16**(E158): Published 2019 Dec 5. https://doi.org/10.5888/pcd16.190212

19 Davis-Floyd, R.E. and C.F. Sargent, *Childbirth and authoritative knowledge: Cross-cultural perspectives.* 1997: University of California Press, Oakland.

20 Regmi, K., et al., *Decentralization and district health services in Nepal: Understanding the views of service users and service providers.* Journal of Public Health, 2010. **32**(3): p. 406–417.

21 Bhandari, A., M. Gordon, and G. Shakya, *Reducing maternal mortality in Nepal.* BJOG: An International Journal of Obstetrics and Gynaecology, 2011. **118**(s2): p. 26–30.

22 Janevic, T., et al., *Neighborhood deprivation and adverse birth outcomes among diverse ethnic groups.* Annals of Epidemiology, 2010. **20**(6): p. 445–451.

23 Liu, N., et al., *Neighbourhood family income and adverse birth outcomes among singleton deliveries.* Journal of Obstetrics and Gynaecology Canada, 2010. **32**(11): p. 1042–1048.

24 Labonte, R., *Heart health inequalities in Canada: Modules, theory and planning.* Health Promotion International, 1992. **7**(2): p. 119–128.

25 Marmot, M. and R. Bell, *Health equity and development: The commission on social determinants of health.* European Review, 2010. **18**(1): p. 1.

26 World Health Organisation, *Trends in maternal mortality 2000 to 2017: Estimates by WHO, UNICEF.* UNFPA, World Bank Group and the United Nations Population Division. Geneva. Retrieved April, 2019. **1**: p. 2020.

27 Wagle, R.R., S. Sabroe, and B.B. Nielsen, *Socioeconomic and physical distance to the maternity hospital as predictors for place of delivery: An observation study from Nepal.* BMC Pregnancy and Childbirth, 2004. **4**(1): p. 8.

28 Bhutta, Z.A. and M. Chopra, *The countdown for 2015: What lies ahead?* The Lancet, 2012. **380**(9848): p. 1125–1127.

29 Bhutta, Z.A., et al., *Countdown to 2015 decade report (2000–10): Taking stock of maternal, newborn, and child survival.* The Lancet, 2010. **375**(9730): p. 2032–2044.

30 Bhutta, Z.A., et al., *Maternal and child health: Is South Asia ready for change?* British Medical Journal, 2004. **328**(7443): p. 816–819.

31 Boerma, T., et al., *Countdown to 2030: Tracking progress towards universal coverage for reproductive, maternal, newborn, and child health.* The Lancet, 2018. **391**(10129): p. 1538–1548.

32 Blas, E. and A.S. Kurup, *Equity, social determinants and public health programmes.* 2010: World Health Organization, Geneva.

33 Blas, E., et al., *Social determinants approaches to public health: From concept to practice.* 2011: World Health Organization, Geneva.

34 Langlois, É.V., et al., *Protocol for a systematic review on inequalities in postnatal care services utilization in low-and middle-income countries.* Systematic Reviews, 2013. **2**(1): p. 55.

35 Hong, R. and R. Them, *Inequality in access to health care in Cambodia: Socioeconomically disadvantaged women giving birth at home assisted by unskilled birth attendants.* Asia Pacific Journal of Public Health, 2015. **27**(2): p. 1039–1049.

36 Morrison, J., et al., *Utilization and management of maternal and child health funds in rural Nepal.* Community Development Journal, 2010. **45**(1): p. 75–89.

37 Morrison, J., et al., *Community mobilisation and health management committee strengthening to increase birth attendance by trained health workers in rural Makwanpur, Nepal: Study protocol for a cluster randomised controlled trial.* Trials, 2011. **12**(1): p. 128.

38 Petchesky, R.P., *Global prescriptions: Gendering health and human rights.* 2003: Zed Books, London.

39 Smith, S.L. and S. Neupane, *Factors in health initiative success: Learning from Nepal's newborn survival initiative.* Social Science and Medicine, 2011. **72**(4): p. 568–575.

40 Freire, P., *Pedagogy of the oppressed.* 2018: Bloomsbury Publishing, London.

41 Freire, P. and A.M.A. Freire, *Pedagogy of hope: Reliving pedagogy of the oppressed.* 2004: A & C Black, London.

42 Shor, I. and P. Freire, *A pedagogy for liberation: Dialogues on transforming education.* 1987: Greenwood Publishing Group, Westport.

43 Young, I.M., *Five faces of oppression. Rethinking power.* 2014: State University of New York Press, New York.

44 Heath, R.G., *Rethinking community collaboration through a dialogic lens: Creativity, democracy, and diversity in community organizing.* Management Communication Quarterly, 2007. **21**(2): p. 145–171.

45 Malla, D., et al., *Achieving millennium development goals 4 and 5 in Nepal.* BJOG: An International Journal of Obstetrics and Gynaecology, 2011. **118**: p. 60–68.

46 Powell-Jackson, T. and K. Hanson, *Financial incentives for maternal health: Impact of a national programme in Nepal.* Journal of Health Economics, 2012. **31**(1): p. 271–284.

47 Witter, S., et al., *The national free delivery policy in Nepal: Early evidence of its effects on health facilities.* Health Policy and Planning, 2011. **26**(2): p. 84–91.

48 Adam, T., et al., *Cost effectiveness analysis of strategies for maternal and neonatal health in developing countries.* British Medical Journal, 2005. **331**(7525): p. 1107.

49 Neupane, D. and G. Gulis, *Comment on: Attracting and retaining doctors in rural Nepal.* Rural and Remote Health. 2010. **10**(3): p. 1420.

50 Wikler, D., *Personal and social responsibility for health.* Ethics and International Affairs, 2002. **16**(2): p. 47–55.

51 Crawford, R., *Individual responsibility and health politics* in the Sociology of Health and Illness, 1986: St. Martin's Press, New York.

52 Mittelmark, M.B., *Promoting social responsibility for health: Health impact assessment and healthy public policy at the community level.* Health Promotion International, 2001. **16**(3): p. 269.

53 Grodin, M.A., S. Gruskin, and J.M. Mann, *Health and human rights: A reader.* 1999: Routledge, London.

54 Gruskin, S., et al., *Using human rights to improve maternal and neonatal health: History, connections and a proposed practical approach.* Bulletin of the World Health Organization, 2008. **86**: p. 589–593.

7 Insights for policy and practice
The WCEC model of childbirth

Introduction

Childbirth is an ongoing part of everyday life for women living in remote mountains of Nepal. This research aimed to address a gap in the evidence to date and to uncover local voices to more fully understand the factors that have an impact on the childbirth experiences of women. In doing so, it intended to provide insight into what may contribute to reducing the unacceptably high numbers of maternal and newborn deaths in the region. This research identified a wide range of diverging but intertwining factors which influenced childbirth in the mountains. Childbirth experiences of women in remote communities are influenced by their embedded culture, tradition, knowledge, belief system, social norms and spirituality [1].

There is a perception that women in remote mountains are traditionally forced to give birth in the Goth and to spend their "polluted" postnatal days creating the risk of neonatal infection [2–5]. However, this research confirmed that women have more agency than that, and it is a tradition they choose to adopt for their safety. Although the belief in supernatural powers during childbirth is not often discussed regarding other cultures [6–8], the cultural construct of childbirth was a significant factor contributing to the perception safety for remote mountain women. In their perspective, even medicine and technology did not supersede their belief in the power of God to ensure the survival of mother and baby during the birth. In this situation, breaking their connection to this spiritual relationship created a threat to the safety of childbirth.

This research demonstrated a tension between how the concept of risk is constructed in the medical model and the way the concept of safety is constructed in the traditional–cultural model of childbirth. The medical model imposes that there is a risk associated with giving birth in the Goth and recommends bringing women to the hospital to give birth. However, acting on medical risks contradicts the cultural construction of safety for women, as women preferred to stay in the community and follow childbirth traditions. Nevertheless, women confirmed the lack of medical assistance to manage the risks involved in childbirth locally limiting options to determine safety.

This research further revealed a complex pattern of relationships at the family and societal level. In these relationships, power had a strong influence on the childbirth experiences of the women. Where the family relationship was support-ive, women were more likely to experience safe childbirth. As in other studies [4, 9–14], the role of the mother-in-law and husband were crucial to the birthing experiences of women. Despite the role other family members play in childbirth decisions, embedded power, trust and respect were significant enabling aspects in these relationships. Women trusted the traditional knowledge and support of local care providers in the community more than the medical knowledge and care provided by professionals in the hospital. This shows the power of traditional knowledge and the importance of considering it to ensure safety during childbirth, which is supported and continued through familiarity, respect and understanding.

In the remote mountain communities, community-based care providers were able to develop a shared understanding and were respectful towards the women and were therefore able to gain respect and trust from the women to help them during childbirth. Health professionals were lacking that trust and respect from the women because they neither show respect towards the women nor their socio-cultural background. Where women were able to develop a trust and gain respect-ful support, they were more comfortable allowing others to make decisions to achieve safe childbirth experiences. In contrast, when there was no trust estab-lished, there was a power exercised over women which created a threat to a safe childbirth experience. This provided a very important insight into healthcare prac-tice, revealing that the medical model is limited in gaining the trust and respect of women, which threatens the management of associated risks.

Despite the continuing efforts of government and non-governmental organisa-tions to increase access to care and resources for rural, remote and marginalised groups in Nepal [15–17], remote mountain women still experience many social, political and structural constraints. More importantly, the inadequate production and supply of food due to adverse climatic conditions made the situation more critical. Difficulties of accessing basic health care added to the complexity. For them, reaching hospital services was not a practical option when they needed medical help. Additionally, there were significant policy and practice gaps such as policy efforts for bringing women to the health institutions to give birth without making services available to them demonstrates the criticality of women's access to resources, opportunities and services.

In similar cross-cultural settings, collaborative planning processes have been successful which brought community, stakeholders, service providers and poli-cymakers together to develop appropriate intervention strategies for childbirth safety [18–21]. Collaborative approaches have contributed to sustaining the trust and relationships in cross-cultural communities and resulted in partnerships to design culturally responsive childbirth services for women. It could further enable to create a supportive environment for remote mountain women to experience safe childbirth and to improve birth outcomes.

The collaborative concept supports the process of bringing women, family members, stakeholders, service providers, politicians and community together to discuss the issues, constraints and possibilities to take locally appropriate actions [22, 23]. On top of this, enabling community participation to address a wide range of determinants impacting birth outcomes allows the government to utilise the local strengths and resources [24–26]. Having a community voice both in structures and agencies is important for women because their involvement in decision-making processes has not yet been established and appreciated [1, 27]. Developing women's capacity to negotiate for changes and the resources they require to gain safe childbirth experiences is critical for both policy and practice [28]. Utilising the social determinants approach to health helps to understand the complexities including the social, political, economic, environmental and cultural factors that have a strong impact on childbirth experiences of women.

A socio-environmental approach to health emphasised the role of collaboration in decision-making process for improved perceptions of safety; improved social support structure; a more supportive healthcare system; improved ability for the community and women to determine how resources are used and distributed; and shifts in equity and power that lead to better outcomes [29]. This transformative collaboration not only enables all components critical to childbirth safety to be addressed; it also fosters a supportive environment for women during childbirth [30]. As both cultural and medical approaches have their own strengths and limitations, the contributions of these approaches are needed to gain safe, satisfying and empowering childbirth experiences, which is possible through collaboration.

The argument made here is not about deciding between birth in the community or in an institution – it is about ensuring safe birthing experiences in which women are able to use both traditional and medical services. By doing so, women can sustain their childbirth tradition, ensure cultural safety and experience positive birth outcomes. As some women have already shown the power of negotiation in sustaining supportive relationships and maintaining traditional knowledge within the medical environment, it is pertinent to put the collaborative childbirth model into practice. Indeed, ensuring childbirth safety is everyone's responsibility.

The context of childbirth in the mountains is like a jigsaw puzzle for women. There are multiple intertwining factors that create uncertainties about the survival of mothers and babies during childbirth, and to date, there have been no solutions proposed to address these factors effectively. Drawing on insights from this research, I attempt to put the pieces of the puzzle together to propose a collaborative model of childbirth that addresses the related risks and promotes the maternal and newborn survival in complex cross-cultural settings. Instead of debating about the medical risk or cultural safety, the model I propose offers an opportunity to establish services which respect elements of both cultural and medical models.

The WCEC model of childbirth: a way forward

The lived experiences gathered in this research suggest that both cultural practices and medical approaches contribute to enhancing childbirth safety in remote mountain regions of Nepal. In this case, those who hold knowledge about culture and those who hold knowledge about medicine need to come together collaboratively to negotiate a relationship which is complementary, and which enables both knowledge holders to play appropriate roles to promote survival of mothers and babies. However, this collaboration is not possible without a shared understanding and responsibility. Although it is a challenging task to create an environment in which the strengths of divergent ways of thinking come together to enhance childbirth safety in a complex social setting, I am hopeful that a collaborative process will help to guide future policy and practice.

From my conversations with women, family members and other community stakeholders, it became apparent that childbirth in the remote mountains is a complex social experience. To make it a safe, liberating and satisfying experience for women requires a woman-centred and collaborative approach. Drawing key components from this research, I have developed a simple collaborative childbirth model that could be useful not only to improve the childbirth experience of women in remote mountains of Nepal but also in any social and cross-cultural community setting. The WCEC refers to women centred, culturally safe, empowering and collaborative model of childbirth.

Woman centred

A woman-centred approach recognises the influence of family and community and respects socio-cultural circumstances of women in which childbirth occurs. It aims to meet the physical, emotional, psychological, spiritual, social and cultural needs by creating an enabling environment for women to take ownership and control of their childbirth experiences [31–35]. This approach gives power to women to decide where and how they want their childbirth to occur. In doing so, women

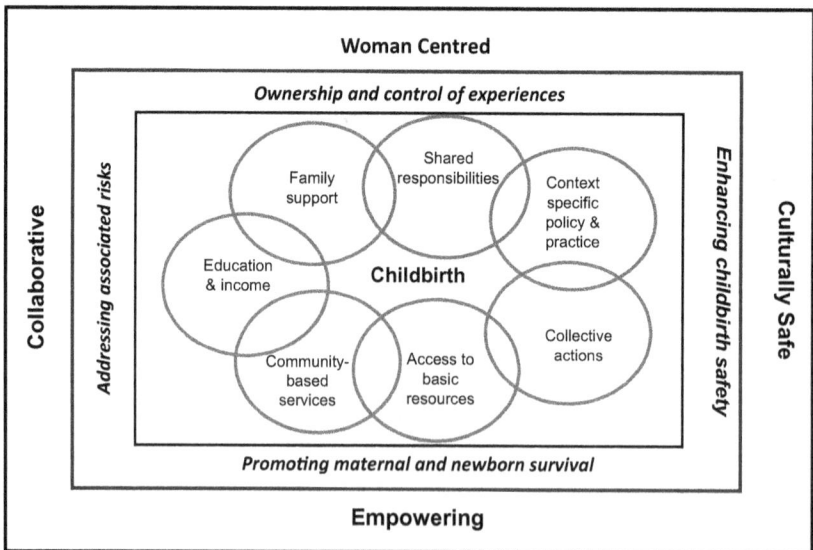

Figure 7.1 The WCEC model of childbirth

can establish an equal partnership with their trusted support person to make childbirth a comfortable, safe, empowering and satisfying experience.

Culturally safe

Maintaining culture, tradition and spirituality was the most important aspect of childbirth for women in the remote mountains. The need to provide culturally safe childbirth support and care for women from cross-cultural communities has consistently been highlighted [36–40]. Women who attended institutional services mentioned the threat they felt for their cultural safety while giving birth and revealed the significance of having a culturally safe environment to make their birthing a positive experience. All care providers, professionals, midwives, clinical staff and other support persons must take women's cultural needs into account while providing care. This further emphasised the need for policymakers to ensure that culturally safe approaches inform the design of programmes and services for women.

Empowering

There is adequate evidence to support the importance of childbirth being an empowering experience for women living in any social circumstances by ensuring women can make choices about when, where and how they would like to give birth [34, 41–44]. Although the decision does not always sit with women, it is pertinent that women have control of the birthing process. In this sense, the decision about childbirth must sit with women whether it is at an institution or at home. Other people and professionals involved in the birthing process should create an enabling environment for women.

Collaborative

Women in this research consistently highlighted the contributions of both cultural and medical models to enhancing childbirth safety. Their survival is possible only through the careful consideration of cultural, medical, social, emotional and spiritual risks in policies, programmes and services. Other studies have described the importance of collaboration in providing care to women [45–49]. The collaborative approach is the underpinning ethos in this model that brings women, family members, community, service providers, support persons, community-based care providers and stakeholders together to design culturally appropriate, medically recommended, physically accessible and socially safe childbirth services could be effective to address associated risks and childbirth-related deaths.

Outcomes of the WCEC model

The middle layer of the model focuses on four outcomes with seven core elements which are critical to women, family members, service providers and the community.

OWNERSHIP AND CONTROL OF EXPERIENCES

Even within collectivist social settings, childbirth is a unique personal experience. Each woman makes the meaning of that experience differently. It is important that women have opportunities to decide how and where they would like to give birth, so they can take ownership and control of their experience. Allowing women to take ownership and control of childbirth experiences has been discussed widely [50–54]. I argue that in a society where childbirth is a collective event, the woman should still be at the centre of that experience, with the contributions of trusted supports to make their childbirth an empowering and satisfying moment. So, giving women the opportunity to take ownership and control of their childbirth experiences should become the priority of both policy and practice.

ADDRESSING ASSOCIATED RISKS

Findings of the current research highlighted the need to address modifiable physical and social risk factors to reduce the prevalence of poor birth outcomes, which is consistent with other evidence [1, 31, 55–58]. Addressing these risks have been particularly significant to the women in the mountains because of the disconnect between medical constructions of risk and the number of social, cultural and spiritual risks associated with childbirth. I strongly urge policy and practice to understand the impacts of all forms of risks and develop strategies to address these appropriately.

ENHANCING CHILDBIRTH SAFETY

The socio-cultural perspective emphasises the significance of safety during childbirth. In practice, what has been evident in the literature that most childbirth interventions focused on enhancing physical safety [59–64]. The notion of safety I am referring to here encompasses the physical, emotional, social, cultural and spiritual dimensions that are critical to women. Importantly, the women in my research were more committed to maintaining social, cultural and spiritual safety, giving only limited attention to their physical and emotional safety. I strongly argue the need to give equal emphasis to all aspects of safety when it comes to childbirth. Thus, promoting childbirth safety should become the overarching outcome of policy and practice.

PROMOTING MATERNAL AND NEWBORN SURVIVAL

Promoting the survival of mothers and babies has long been the focus in South Asia [65–68]; however, countries are still struggling to reduce the deaths in remote areas. Taking appropriate measures to prevent childbirth-related deaths must be an ongoing priority of the government and other sectors. Focusing on factors that are contributing to poor birth outcomes, directly or indirectly, could help to address the existing inequalities in maternal and newborn health. Evidence that emerged in this research suggests the criticality of taking broader social, political and structural determinants into account when developing policies and programmes to promote childbirth-related survival in complex social settings.

Elements of the WCEC model

The inner layer of the model represents the core elements that needs consideration while designing services aiming to promote better outcomes by ensuring child-birth safety of women living in a complex cross-cultural setting.

EDUCATION AND INCOME

SES defines an individual's position within a hierarchical social structure in which education and income are the key indicators of measurement. The link between poor SES and adverse birth outcomes has been widely reported [69–73]. In this study, participants indicated the possibility of education and better economic status to contribute for better childbirth experiences. Where poverty and ignorance played a critical role in making reproductive or childbirth-related decisions for women, focusing on education and income generation activities could enhance the capacity of women to make informed and appropriate decisions around when, where and how childbirth occurs. Investing in education and income generation programmes will help to address a wide range of social, cultural and economic factors that are crucial for childbirth safety.

COMMUNITY-BASED SERVICES

Women suggested that access to community-based services is needed when they experience childbirth-related problems. While social circumstances restrict women from leaving their home to seek medical care, making services available locally would be the best strategy for promoting maternal and newborn survival. It is common that women in rural, remote and cross-cultural communities place high value on childbirth culture, belief and traditions, and that leaving their community to give birth threatens their perception of safety [18, 19, 74–76]. Consequently, women place high importance on the place of birth and prefer giving birth in the community to uphold the sense of security and cultural safety. Several examples provided in this research confirmed the need and significance of community-based services to provide safe childbirth experiences.

FAMILY SUPPORTS

Childbirth is a natural and joyful event for most women, but for those living in a complex social environment, the experience becomes challenging to get through alone. In all social settings, continuous support from family has been crucial to making childbirth a positive experience for women [14, 77–80]. Women appreciated the significant role that family members played while making childbirth-related decisions in this study. In most instances, the support family provided contributed to an enhanced perception of safety and led to the improved birth outcomes. This opens the opportunity to develop a family-centred educational programme on safe pregnancy, childbirth and postnatal experiences, to address associated risks more effectively. This is especially important for remote mountain women whose responsibility towards family overshadows their childbirth needs, involving family to provide the required support must be intrinsic to policy and practice.

ACCESS TO BASIC RESOURCES

Most women living in poverty experience poor birth outcomes due to limited access to information, support, opportunities, services and resources to meet the survival needs [81]. There is a direct link between poverty and birth outcomes where poor women are less likely to use the services and are more likely to experience poor pregnancy and birth outcomes [82–84]. For remote mountain women, the lack of basic health care available, persistent food insecurity and difficulties accessing specialised childbirth services when problems arise have always been critical. Not having access to basic resources for survival is a violation of human rights which these women raised seriously. To address the higher numbers of childbirth-related deaths in socio-economically vulnerable communities, it is important to provide women with access to the basic resources required for everyday life [81, 85, 86]. Geographic remoteness further disadvantaged women with the burden of managing everyday food needs for families. This calls for an effort by governments to ensure access to food, basic health services, information and other opportunities for women locally.

SHARED RESPONSIBILITIES

Childbirth is not only a woman's business. Providing a safer environment for giving birth should become everyone's responsibility, so we can address the factors that impact childbirth safety effectively. The notion of shared responsibilities entails cross-sectoral collaboration and invites policymakers, practitioners, stakeholders, leaders, community, family members, service providers and women to work together to design, deliver and sustain community-based childbirth services [87–92]. While there are various socio-cultural factors influencing the way that women experience childbirth, everyone in the society and family has a part to play. This research confirmed that changing the landscape of maternal and newborn health in the remote mountains is only possible when the government, healthcare system and community take accountability to ensure childbirth safety. The component of shared responsibilities must reflect across policy and practice.

COLLECTIVE ACTIONS

Community-based approaches in public health recognise the value of collective actions to create positive change. This applies to childbirth in socially marginalised communities where access to resources and services are problematic and challenging. Evidence suggests that creating an enabling environment for everyone to come together to take actions from their level can generate positive impacts to make childbirth experience safe and empowering for women [93–97]. This research reinforces the need for collective actions to address the wide ranges of social and structural determinants impacting their health, well-being and childbirth. The most critical factors such as ongoing food insecurity, gendered social constructs and chronic poverty are beyond the capacity of the health system alone – only the collective actions taken at every level by all sectors through partnership with the local community can possibly address it.

CONTEXT-SPECIFIC POLICY AND PRACTICE

Childbirth experiences of women vary according to the socio-economic position and the context of the societies. Over the last two decades, socio-economic differences remained the greatest predictor of inequalities in maternal and newborn health outcomes. Despite the efforts made by the government to tackle higher levels of mortality within the country, rural and remote communities are still unable to make expected progress to ensure maternal and newborn survival. There have been consistent attempts to make maternal, newborn and child health a political priority [97–101], but most countries are still struggling with the existing inequalities in birth outcomes. Universal policies and approaches taken by the health systems are not working for vulnerable groups. The gaps in policy and practice to understand and address the corresponding needs for enabling childbirth experience without the uncertainties of survival remain a challenge. It is important to ensure that the policies and practices are reflective of the context of women, family, community and the broader society.

The WCEC model: application to practice

Successful, tailored community-based childbirth service models with a focus on cultural safety have been implemented with Aboriginal and Intuit communities Australia and Canada [19, 20, 102–105]. These examples confirm the cultural and social appropriateness of the approaches taken to address the local needs to make childbirth a safer experience for all women. The success of these services was based on the ability to incorporate the socio-cultural circumstances of women by providing them with access to culturally appropriate information, resources and services, so they can make an informed choice about childbirth. These programmes ensured the cross-sectoral collaboration and community participation in decision-making processes by creating relevant policies, strategies and guidelines to promote childbirth safety [102, 103, 105]. Although the context of remote mountain women in Nepal is different to Aboriginal and Intuit women, there are similarities in terms of how they value culture and tradition with the preference of giving birth within their community setting.

Drawing on insights from the successful implementation of culturally informed childbirth models among Aboriginal women in Australia and Intuit women in Canada [19, 103] and the lived experiences of remote mountain women from Nepal, I propose a few strategies against each component to put the WCEC model into practice. Agreeing with the common view that there is "no one size fits all approach," it is important to take the context of women into account when designing programmes, services and care models. While this is a proposed model for remote, rural and disadvantaged communities but still works across all communities to provide effective and culturally appropriate services.

This model is an impetus for transforming practice by involving women, family members and community in the process enabling them to plan the action required to

Table 7.1 Suggested strategies and examples against each element of model

Elements	Suggested strategies	Practice examples
Education and awareness	General literacy programme	Literacy classes
	Girl's education	Scholarship for girls
	Reproductive health education	Adolescent RH education
	Community education activities	Community workshops
Community-based services	Community-led planning	Community birthing centre
	Local midwife and health workers	Community governance
	Adequate supplies of resources	Flexible and respectful care
	Localised healthcare system	Culturally safe environment
Family supports	Family-centred planning	Respect for family involvement
	Family education programme	Develop resources for families
	Capacity building of family	Enabling environment for family
	Continuity of care model	Role of family as care providers
Access to basic resources	Food security plan	Localised food production and supplies
	Communication and transport measures	Provision of transport for emergency referral
	Localised basic healthcare system	Resourced healthcare centre
	Culturally appropriate information and support	Trained healthcare providers
Shared responsibilities	Shared care model for childbirth	Community-owned services
	Collaborative planning process	Shared accountability and responses
	Multidisciplinary approach	Equitable distribution of resources
	Community-controlled governance	Shared understanding and supports
Collective actions	Collective impact approach	Collective impact process
	Shared action plan	Community-based actions
	Monitoring and evaluation plan	Ongoing documentation
	Reporting and accountability framework	Celebration of achievements
Context specific policy and practice	Remote and rural health policy	Addressing social determinants
	Cultural competency framework	Culturally competent workforce
	Culturally responsive childbirth service	Welcoming and respectful service environment
	Community outreach and home care	Quality of care guidelines
	Cultural safety framework	Cultural safety training to staff

make necessary changes. This shed lights on the need for understanding the socio-cultural dimensions of women, their experiences and preferences to design specific policy and practice for the reduction of maternal, perinatal and newborn mortality.

Underpinning principles of the WCEC model

A framework comprising spiritual, cultural, social and emotional well-being, environmental and economic determinants must be utilised to improve maternal, perinatal and newborn health outcomes in low resource settings. This model provides a critical foundation for the development of appropriate policies and strategies for cross-cultural and disadvantaged community settings to provide safe and liberating childbirth experiences for women based on the following principles:

1   The WCEC model places the woman at the centre of her own care, with the support from professionals, family members and other people in the community to meet cultural, emotional, psychosocial and clinical needs.
2   Collaboration enables women to choose where and how they would like to experience childbirth, taking their socio-cultural circumstances into account to ensure safety.
3   Collaborative processes ensure women have access to culturally and socially appropriate information to make informed decisions about pregnancy and childbirth.
4   Collaboration with women, healthcare providers, decision makers, family members, stakeholders and community help to establish an inclusive, trusting, respectful and culturally safe communication strategy.
5   The WCEC framework is underpinned by principles of safety and quality allowing both culture and medicine to work together to promote health outcomes for mothers and babies.
6   Collaboration aims to enhance the continuity of care throughout pregnancy, birth and the early postnatal period by building the capacity of the family, community support person and other local care providers to maximise the chances of maternal, perinatal and newborn survival.
7   The collaborative practice helps to build trust and mutual respect by fostering shared accountability for managing risks and promoting safety.
8   Collaboration uses a flexible approach to meet the diverse and emerging needs of women, service environments, communities, professionals and service providers.

Policy consideration areas

All women have access to high quality and culturally safe services in the community setting

The evidence suggests that when women need to leave their homes to receive care due to the lack of availability of services in the community, they may experience adverse health outcomes because of being away from their family and being in a different environment [36, 37, 40]. Childbirth services should be high quality and made culturally and socially accessible to women in their communities [106]. Continuous training for health professionals, appropriate infrastructure and equipment, allocation of enough financial and technical resources, localised governance structures for service management and ongoing monitoring of services could help to ensure that women have access to high quality and culturally safe services in the community.

Socio-cultural circumstances of women are taken into the consideration while designing and providing childbirth services

Women living in complex socio-cultural settings have distinct needs in terms of their culture, social system, health belief, geographic features, resources, knowledge and healthcare practice, and are most likely to experience multiple barriers to access services [3, 107–109]. The local contexts of women must be considered when designing and providing health services, so that the care provided is culturally appropriate and responsive to their needs [110–112]. This could be achieved by engaging service providers, including midwives, physicians, nurses and other health professionals, stakeholders, service planners, community and women representatives in planning, implementation and evaluation of all services.

Professionals working in complex socio-cultural settings are supported with additional resources, training and professional development opportunities

All professionals should receive training about the collaborative childbirth model to make sure that women have equitable access to culturally safe care in the community [45, 47, 48]. There should be additional resources and funding allocated to support these professionals to live and work locally in the community, so they can provide continuity of care throughout the pregnancy, childbirth and postnatal period. A mechanism for cross-sectoral collaboration to shift healthcare delivery from the regional to local level should be in place to address the broader social determinants [98, 101]. Recruiting young women from the communities to train them to be midwives could be beneficial in the long-term, so women are able to receive care in the community by a trusted person. This might take longer to implement, so it is important to have strategies to retain a broad range of healthcare providers within communities to ensure the ongoing provision of quality of care.

Service delivery framework reflects the realities of the community, incorporates emerging evidence and maintains relevance to the practice environment

The service delivery framework should consider the principles of continuity of care, informed choice, woman-centred care, cultural safety and making childbirth a liberating experience for women [19, 103–105]. The service delivery model should reflect what women want, when women want the care and how women want the care to be provided to them [42]. While considering women's choices, the quality of care provided to women should not be compromised due to socio-cultural circumstances [20]. This could be achieved by investing enough resources to address the socio-cultural needs of the population, which is critical to their health and well-being.

All women of reproductive age are empowered with better access to information, education, resources and services to maintain their health and well-being

Growing evidence internationally indicates that giving reproductive aged girls and women access to information, education, resources and services makes a significant difference to health outcomes [41]. This enables all women to make decisions about marriage and pregnancy when they are physically and emotionally mature. It is critical to provide women with choices to decide where, when and how they would like to give birth, making sure the cultural, emotional and physical aspects of childbirth safety are considered [34, 42]. This will help to minimise the impacts of young age marriage and pregnancy in birth outcomes and contribute to reducing the related morbidities and mortalities in the community [113]. Education and empowerment will further assist women to gain better social status to engage in broader social, economic and political opportunities.

Community leadership and collaborative partnerships are taken as the priorities for sustained and improved health outcomes for everyone

Using the concept of PHC, community leadership and collaborative partnerships are key pillars of the health system, which could help to identify local needs, resources and solutions to address the complex determinants leading to poor outcomes [114, 115]. Embedding community leadership and collaborative partnerships as policy priorities across all sectors generates a sense of trust, ownership and agency in the community and helps to address the social and structural issues impacting the whole population [90, 95]. Engaging multiple sectors and the community in collaboration for planning, delivering and evaluating services and programmes is a cost-effective way to promote health outcomes in low resource settings [87]. Following the notion of health is everyone's responsibility [97], a collaborative approach helps to create collective impacts in the community.

Ongoing monitoring and evaluation with both quantitative and qualitative measures are in place to assess the changes in maternal, perinatal and newborn health outcomes

Ongoing monitoring and evaluation are an essential part of any health system, to ensure that all women receive the right care, at the right time, in the right place and by the right people [98, 116, 117]. This enables interested stakeholders to measure the impacts of the policies and strategies that are in place and to determine whether women have gained safer childbirth experiences in the community [118, 119]. The outcomes can be measured using both quantitative and qualitative indicators to understand trends and experiences with the services. This will help governments to determine where further resources and support should be allocated to improve outcomes on a population level, and what other measures are required to address the maternal, perinatal and newborn health issues in socially complex settings.

Context-specific strategies are in place to cater the needs of rural and remote communities

Within broader policy initiatives, the government should develop context-specific strategies to address the issues that rural and remote communities face in terms of accessing and utilising health services [120–122]. There should be a concerted effort on several fronts targeting the appropriate design, delivery and structure of services, enhancing communication and infrastructure, supporting the health workforce, building community capacity and enabling women to make informed decisions [123, 124]. This will help to reduce the inequalities in maternal, perinatal and newborn health outcomes that countries and regions are experiencing currently [125, 126]. Strategic outcome areas may include improved access to appropriate, culturally safe and comprehensive health care; effective, accessible, community-based and sustainable maternity services; an appropriate, skilled, culturally competent and well-supported health workforce; a collaborative health service planning and policy development process; strong and collaborative leadership, partnerships, governance and accountability; and standardised data collection, monitoring and reporting system.

Conclusion

The social environment that women give birth has significant influence on perception of safety, emotional well-being and the birth outcomes. Although remote mountain women accept pregnancy and childbirth as everyday part of their life, their choices and options are compromised due to the social circumstances of their living. When childbirth is impacted by complex social and cultural factors, the only hope for making that experience safe and empowering is by giving women access to resources, services and authority to make decisions.

The collaborative model of childbirth is designed to promote the active engagement of various sectors, community, family and women in designing and providing high-quality care that is tailored to meet the needs of women prior to, during and after childbirth. The WCEC model incorporates evidence from research based on the notion that childbirth services should be woman-centred, culturally safe, empowering and collaborative to enable improved access, choice and appropriateness of services to all women in the community.

The proposed model provides a guiding framework for planning and providing context specific services to promote the maternal, perinatal and newborn health outcomes not only in low resource, socially complex and disadvantaged communities, as well as for informing policy and practice in cross-cultural settings. Taking a collaborative approach with sustained partnerships, community leadership, engagement of all sectors and participation of community, family and women in decision-making process could help to address the broader social and structural determinants to ensure that all women have access to socially appropriate, culturally safe and high-quality care for improved health and well-being outcomes.

References

1 Kaphle, S., H. Hancock, and L.A. Newman, *Childbirth traditions and cultural perceptions of safety in Nepal: Critical spaces to ensure the survival of mothers and newborns in remote mountain villages.* Midwifery, 2013. **29**(10): p. 1173–1181.

2 Ahmed, M., et al., *Utilization of rural maternity delivery services in Nawalparasi and Kapilvastu District: A Qualitative Study.* Journal of College of Medical Sciences-Nepal, 2010. **6**(3): p. 29–36.

3 Ahmed, S., et al., *Economic status, education and empowerment: Implications for maternal health service utilization in developing countries.* PloS One, 2010. **5**(6).

4 Regmi, K. *Childbirth practices in Nepal: A review of models for reducing adverse outcomes.* International Journal of Gynaecology and Obstetrics, 2009 **10**(9): p. 321.

5 Thapa, N., et al., *High-risk childbirth practices in remote Nepal and their determinants.* Women and Health, 2001. **31**(4): p. 83–97.

6 Belousova, E., *The Preservation of National childbirth Traditions in the Russian homebirth community.* FOLKLORICA-Journal of the Slavic, East European, and Eurasian Folklore Association, 2002. **7**(2).

7 Lori, J.R. and J.S. Boyle, *Cultural childbirth practices, beliefs, and traditions in post-conflict Liberia.* Health Care for Women International, 2011. **32**(6): p. 454–473.

8 Marak, Q., *Supernatural beliefs connected with childbirth among the garos of Assam.* The Oriental Anthropologist, 2004. **4**(2): p. 186–190.

9 Acharya, P.P. and D. Rimal, Pregnancy and childbirth in Nepal: Women's role and decision-making power, in *Childbirth across Cultures.* 2009: Springer, New York. p. 137–144.

10 Brunson, J., *Confronting maternal mortality, controlling birth in Nepal: The gendered politics of receiving biomedical care at birth.* Social Science and Medicine, 2010. **71**(10): p. 1719–1727.

11 Basnyat, I., *Beyond biomedicine: Health through social and cultural understanding.* Nursing Inquiry, 2011. **18**(2): p. 123–134.

12 Dhakal, S., et al., *Skilled care at birth among rural women in Nepal: Practice and challenges.* Journal of Health, Population, and Nutrition, 2011. **29**(4): p. 371.

13 Simkhada, B., M.A. Porter, and E.R. Van Teijlingen, *The role of mothers-in-law in antenatal care decision-making in Nepal: A qualitative study.* BMC Pregnancy and Childbirth, 2010. **10**(1): p. 34.

14 Lewis, S., A. Lee, and P. Simkhada, *The role of husbands in maternal health and safe childbirth in rural Nepal: A qualitative study.* BMC Pregnancy and Childbirth, 2015. **15**(1): p. 162.

15 Morrison, J., et al., *Utilization and management of maternal and child health funds in rural Nepal.* Community Development Journal, 2010. **45**(1): p. 75–89.

16 Morrison, J., et al., *Community mobilisation and health management committee strengthening to increase birth attendance by trained health workers in rural Makwanpur, Nepal: Study protocol for a cluster randomised controlled trial.* Trials, 2011. **12**(1): p. 128.

17 Powell-Jackson, T., et al., *The experiences of districts in implementing a national incentive programme to promote safe delivery in Nepal.* BMC Health Services Research, 2009. **9**(1): p. 97.

18 Douglas, V.K., *The Inuulitsivik maternities: Culturally appropriate midwifery and epistemological accommodation.* Nursing inquiry, 2010. **17**(2): p. 111–117.

19 Douglas, V.K., *The Rankin Inlet birthing centre: Community midwifery in the Inuit context.* International Journal of Circumpolar Health, 2011. **70**(2): p. 178–185.

20 Kildea, S., et al., *Birthing on country (in our community): A case study of engaging stakeholders and developing a best-practice Indigenous maternity service in an urban setting.* Australian Health Review, 2018. **42**(2): p. 230–238.

21 Sarmiento, I., et al., *Indigenous factors relevant for safe birth in cultural safety among Nancue ñomndaa communities in Guerrero, Mexico. Protocol of a study based on conversations.* International Journal of Indigenous Health, 2019. **14**(2): p. 7–18.

22 Shor, I. and P. Freire, *A pedagogy for liberation: Dialogues on transforming education.* 1987: Greenwood Publishing Group, Westport.

23 Heath, R.G., *Rethinking community collaboration through a dialogic lens: Creativity, democracy, and diversity in community organizing.* Management Communication Quarterly, 2007. **21**(2): p. 145–171.

24 Blas, E. and A.S. Kurup, *Equity, social determinants and public health programmes.* 2010: World Health Organization, Geneva.

25 Blas, E., et al., *Social determinants approaches to public health: From concept to practice.* 2011: World Health Organization, Geneva.

26 Freeman, T., et al., *Reaching those with the greatest need: How Australian primary health care service managers, practitioners and funders understand and respond to health inequity.* Australian Journal of Primary Health, 2011. **17**(4): p. 355–361.

27 Gargioni, G. and M. Raviglione, *The principles of primary health care and social justice.* Journal of Medicine and the Person, 2009. **7**(2): p. 103.

28 Kahssay, H.M., P. Oakley, and W.H. Organization, *Community involvement in health development: A review of the concept and practice.* 1999: World Health Organization, Geneva.

29 Labonte, R., *Heart health inequalities in Canada: Modules, theory and planning.* Health Promotion International, 1992. **7**(2): p. 119–128.

30 Young, I.M., *Justice and the politics of difference.* 2011: Princeton University Press, Princeton.

31 Berg, M., Ó.A. Ólafsdóttir, and I. Lundgren, *A midwifery model of woman-centred childbirth care – In Swedish and Icelandic settings.* Sexual and Reproductive Healthcare, 2012. **3**(2): p. 79–87.

32 Hunter, A., et al., *Woman-centred care during pregnancy and birth in Ireland: Thematic analysis of women's and clinicians' experiences.* BMC Pregnancy and Childbirth, 2017. **17**(1): p. 1–11.

33 Leap, N., *Woman-centred or women-centred care: Does it matter?* British Journal of Midwifery, 2009. **17**(1): p. 12–16.

34 Maputle, M.S., *A woman-centred childbirth model.* Journal of Interdisciplinary Health Sciences, 2010. **15**(1): p. 1–8.

35 Maputle, M.S. and H. Donavon, *Woman-centred care in childbirth: A concept analysis (part 1).* Curationis, 2013. **36**(1): p. 1–8.

36 Crowther, S. and J. Hall, *Spirituality and spiritual care in and around childbirth.* Women and Birth, 2015. **28**(2): p. 173–178.

37 Kildea, S. and M. Wardaguga, Childbirth in Australia: Aboriginal and Torres Strait islander women, in *Childbirth across Cultures.* 2009: Springer, New York. p. 275–286.

38 Kim, S.H., K.W. Kim, and K.E. Bae, *Experiences of nurses who provide childbirth care for women with multi-cultural background.* Journal of Korean Public Health Nursing, 2014. **28**(1): p. 87–101.

39 Kruske, S., S. Kildea, and L. Barclay, *Cultural safety and maternity care for Aboriginal and Torres Strait Islander Australians.* Women and Birth, 2006. **19**(3): p. 73–77.

40 Riggs, E., et al., *Cultural safety and belonging for refugee background women attending group pregnancy care: An Australian qualitative study.* Birth, 2017. **44**(2): p. 145–152.

41 Bell, K.M., *Centering pregnancy: Changing the system, empowering women and strengthening families.* International Journal of Childbirth Education, 2012. **27**(1): p. 70.

42 Lazarus, E., What do women want? Issues of choice, control, and class in American pregnancy and childbirth, in *Childbirth and authoritative knowledge: Cross-cultural perspectives.* 1997: University of California Press, Oakland. p. 132–158.

43 Lundgren, I., *Swedish women's experience of childbirth 2 years after birth.* Midwifery, 2005. **21**(4): p. 346–354.

44 Ulfsdottir, H., et al., *Like an empowering micro-home: A qualitative study of women's experience of giving birth in water.* Midwifery, 2018. **67**: p. 26–31.

45 Downe, S., K. Finlayson, and A. Fleming, *Creating a collaborative culture in maternity care.* Journal of Midwifery and Women's Health, 2010. **55**(3): p. 250–254.

46 Harris, S.J., et al., *Effect of a collaborative interdisciplinary maternity care program on perinatal outcomes.* CMAJ, 2012. **184**(17): p. 1885–1892.

47 Kermode, M., et al., *Walking together: Towards a collaborative model for maternal health care in pastoralist communities of Laikipia and Samburu, Kenya.* Maternal and Child Health Journal, 2017. **21**(10): p. 1867–1873.

48 Pecci, C.C., et al., *The birth of a collaborative model: Obstetricians, midwives, and family physicians.* Obstetrics and Gynaecology Clinics, 2012. **39**(3): p. 323–334.

49 Vogt, S.E., K.S.d. Silva, and M.A.B. Dias, *Comparison of childbirth care models in public hospitals, Brazil.* Revista de Saude Publica, 2014. **48**: p. 304–313.

50 Cook, K. and C. Loomis, *The impact of choice and control on women's childbirth experiences.* The Journal of Perinatal Education, 2012. **21**(3): p. 158–168.

51 Jomeen, J., *Choice, control and contemporary childbirth: Understanding through women's stories.* 2010: Radcliffe Publishing, London.

52 Malacrida, C. and T. Boulton, *Women's perceptions of childbirth "choices" competing discourses of motherhood, sexuality, and selflessness.* Gender and Society, 2012. **26**(5): p. 748–772.

53 Meyer, S., *Control in childbirth: A concept analysis and synthesis.* Journal of Advanced Nursing, 2013. **69**(1): p. 218–228.

54 Snowden, A., et al., *Concurrent analysis of choice and control in childbirth.* BMC Pregnancy and Childbirth, 2011. **11**(1): p. 40.

55 Chadwick, R.J. and D. Foster, *Negotiating risky bodies: Childbirth and constructions of risk.* Health, Risk and Society, 2014. **16**(1): p. 68–83.

56   Coxon, K., et al., *Reconceptualising risk in childbirth.* Midwifery, 2016. **38**: p. 1–5. https://doi.org/10.1016/j.midw.2016.05.012

57   Lane, K., *Pluralist risk cultures: The sociology of childbirth in Vanuatu.* Health, Risk and Society, 2015. **17**(5–6): p. 349–367.

58   Maffi, I. and S. Gouilhers, *Conceiving of risk in childbirth: Obstetric discourses, medical management and cultural expectations in Switzerland and Jordan.* Health, Risk and Society, 2019. **21**(3–4): p. 185–206. https://doi.org/10.1080/13698575.2015. 1096326

59   DeJong, J., et al., *The safety and quality of childbirth in the context of health systems: Mapping maternal health provision in Lebanon.* Midwifery, 2010. **26**(5): p. 549–557.

60   Lothian, J.A., *Risk, safety, and choice in childbirth.* The Journal of Perinatal Education, 2012. **21**(1): p. 45–47.

61   Patabendige, M. and H. Senanayake, *Implementation of the WHO safe childbirth checklist program at a tertiary care setting in Sri Lanka: A developing country experience.* BMC Pregnancy and Childbirth, 2015. **15**(1): p. 12.

62   Semrau, K.E., et al., *Effectiveness of the WHO Safe Childbirth Checklist program in reducing severe maternal, foetal, and newborn harm in Uttar Pradesh, India: Study protocol for a matched-pair, cluster-randomized controlled trial.* Trials, 2016. **17**(1): p. 1–10.

63   Spector, J.M., et al., *Improving quality of care for maternal and newborn health: Prospective pilot study of the WHO safe childbirth checklist program.* PloS One, 2012. **7**(5): p. 351–361.

64   Vedam, S., et al., *The mothers on respect (MOR) index: Measuring quality, safety, and human rights in childbirth.* Social Science and Medicine – Population Health, 2017. **3**: p. 201–210. https://doi.org/10.1016/j.ssmph.2017.01.005

65   Bhutta, Z.A., et al., *Maternal and child health: Is South Asia ready for change?* British Medical Journal, 2004. **328**(7443): p. 816–819.

66   Nair, N., et al., *Improving newborn survival in low-income countries: Community-based approaches and lessons from South Asia.* PLoS Med, 2010. **7**(4): p. e1000246.

67   Paul, V.K. The current state of newborn health in low income countries and the way forward, in *Seminars in foetal and neonatal medicine.* 2006: Elsevier, Amsterdam.

68   Requejo, J.H., et al., *Regional collaborations as a way forward for maternal, newborn and child health: The South Asian healthcare professional workshop.* Journal of Health, Population, and Nutrition, 2010. **28**(5): p. 417.

69   Blumenshine, P., et al., *Socioeconomic disparities in adverse birth outcomes: A systematic review.* American Journal of Preventive Medicine, 2010. **39**(3): p. 263–272.

70   Campbell, E.E., et al., *Socioeconomic status and adverse birth outcomes: A population-based Canadian sample.* Journal of Biosocial Science, 2018. **50**(1): p. 102–113.

71   Dominguez, T.P., *Adverse birth outcomes in African American women: The social context of persistent reproductive disadvantage.* Social Work in Public Health, 2011. **26**(1): p. 3–16.

72   Magadi, M., N. Madise, and I. Diamond, *Factors associated with unfavourable birth outcomes in Kenya.* Journal of Biosocial Science, 2001. **33**(2): p. 199–210.

73   Meng, G., M.E. Thompson, and G.B. Hall, *Pathways of neighbourhood-level socioeconomic determinants of adverse birth outcomes.* International Journal of Health Geographics, 2013. **12**(1): p. 1–16.

74   Ireland, S., et al., *Niyith Nniyith Watmam (the quiet story): Exploring the experiences of Aboriginal women who give birth in their remote community.* Midwifery, 2011. **27**(5): p. 634–641.

75   Mahato, P.K., et al., *Birthing centres in Nepal: Recent developments, obstacles and opportunities*. Journal of Asian Midwives, 2016. **3**(1): p. 18–30.

76   Skye, A.D., *Aboriginal midwifery: A model for change*. Journal of Aboriginal Health, 2010. **6**(1).

77   Benza, S. and P. Liamputtong, *Pregnancy, childbirth and motherhood: A meta-synthesis of the lived experiences of immigrant women*. Midwifery, 2014. **30**(6): p. 575–584.

78   Hodnett, E.D., et al., *Continuous support for women during childbirth*. Cochrane Database of Systematic Reviews, 2013(7).

79   Webster, J., et al., *Quality of life and depression following childbirth: Impact of social support*. Midwifery, 2011. **27**(5): p. 745–749.

80   XIE, R.H., et al., *Prenatal family support, postnatal family support and postpartum depression*. Australian and New Zealand Journal of Obstetrics and Gynaecology, 2010. **50**(4): p. 340–345.

81   Izugbara, C.O. and D.P. Ngilangwa, *Women, poverty and adverse maternal outcomes in Nairobi, Kenya*. BMC Women's Health, 2010. **10**(1): p. 1–8.

82   Khatri, R.B., et al., *Barriers to utilization of childbirth services of a rural birthing center in Nepal: A qualitative study*. PloS One, 2017. **12**(5): p. 177–189.

83   Patel, V., M. Rodrigues, and N. DeSouza, *Gender, poverty, and postnatal depression: A study of mothers in Goa, India*. American journal of Psychiatry, 2002. **159**(1): p. 43–47.

84   Wong, K.L., L. Benova, and O.M. Campbell, *A look back on how far to walk: Systematic review and meta-analysis of physical access to skilled care for childbirth in sub-Saharan Africa*. PloS One, 2017. **12**(9): p. 184–196.

85   Barbieri, P. and R. Bozzon, *Welfare, labour market deregulation and households' poverty risks: An analysis of the risk of entering poverty at childbirth in different European welfare clusters*. Journal of European Social Policy, 2016. **26**(2): p. 99–123.

86   Fogliati, P., et al., *How can childbirth care for the rural poor be improved? A contribution from spatial modelling in rural Tanzania*. PloS One, 2015. **10**(9): p. 139–148.

87   Adeleye, O.A. and A.N. Ofili, *Strengthening intersectoral collaboration for primary health care in developing countries: Can the health sector play broader roles?* Journal of Environmental and Public Health, 2010. https://doi.org/10.1155/2010/272896

88   Adongo, P.B., et al., *The role of community-based health planning and services strategy in involving males in the provision of family planning services: A qualitative study in Southern Ghana*. Reproductive Health, 2013. **10**(1): p. 1–15.

89   August, F., et al., *Community health workers can improve male involvement in maternal health: Evidence from rural Tanzania*. Global Health Action, 2016. **9**(1): p. 30064.

90   Awoonor-Williams, J.K., et al., *Lessons learned from scaling up a community-based health program in the Upper East Region of northern Ghana*. Global Health: Science and Practice, 2013. **1**(1): p. 117–133.

91   Possamai-Inesedy, A., *Confining risk: Choice and responsibility in childbirth in a risk society*. Health Sociology Review, 2006. **15**(4): p. 406–414.

92   Yargawa, J. and J. Leonardi-Bee, *Male involvement and maternal health outcomes: Systematic review and meta-analysis*. Journal of Epidemiology Community Health, 2015. **69**(6): p. 604–612.

93   Mafuta, E.M., et al., *Social accountability for maternal health services in Muanda and Bolenge Health Zones, Democratic Republic of Congo: A situation analysis*. BMC Health Services Research, 2015. **15**(1): p. 514.

94 Prost, A., et al., *Women's groups practising participatory learning and action to improve maternal and newborn health in low-resource settings: A systematic review and meta-analysis*. The Lancet, 2013. **381**(9879): p. 1736–1746.

95 Rosato, M., et al., *Community participation: Lessons for maternal, newborn, and child health*. The Lancet, 2008. **372**(9642): p. 962–971.

96 Saggurti, N., et al., *Effect of health intervention integration within women's self-help groups on collectivization and healthy practices around reproductive, maternal, neonatal and child health in rural India*. PloS One, 2018. **13**(8): p. e0202562.

97 Shiffman, J. and S. Smith, *Generation of political priority for global health initiatives: A framework and case study of maternal mortality*. The Lancet, 2007. **370**(9595): p. 1370–1379.

98 Boerma, T., et al., *Countdown to 2030: Tracking progress towards universal coverage for reproductive, maternal, newborn, and child health*. The Lancet, 2018. **391**(10129): p. 1538–1548.

99 Filippi, V., et al., *Maternal health in poor countries: The broader context and a call for action*. The Lancet, 2006. **368**(9546): p. 1535–1541.

100 Smith, S.L. and J. Shiffman, *Setting the global health agenda: The influence of advocates and ideas on political priority for maternal and newborn survival*. Social Science and Medicine, 2016. **166**: p. 86–93. https://doi.org/10.1016/j.socscimed.2016.08.013

101 Victora, C.G., et al., *Countdown to 2015: A decade of tracking progress for maternal, newborn, and child survival*. The Lancet, 2016. **387**(10032): p. 2049–2059.

102 Barclay, L., et al., *Reconceptualising risk: Perceptions of risk in rural and remote maternity service planning*. Midwifery, 2016. **38**: p. 63–70.

103 Kildea, S., et al., *Implementing birthing on country services for Aboriginal and Torres Strait Islander families: RISE framework*. Women and Birth, 2019. **32**(5): p. 466–475.

104 Olson, R. and C. Couchie, *Returning birth: The politics of midwifery implementation on First Nations reserves in Canada*. Midwifery, 2013. **29**(8): p. 981–987.

105 Roe, Y., et al., *Returning birthing services to communities and Aboriginal control: Aboriginal women of Shoalhaven Illawarra region describe how Birthing on Country is linked to healing*. Journal of Indigenous Wellbeing, 2020. **5**(1): p. 58–71.

106 Mander, S. and Y. Miller, *Perceived safety, quality and cultural competency of maternity care for culturally and linguistically diverse women in Queensland*. Journal of Racial and Ethnic Health Disparities, 2016. **3**(1): p. 83–98.

107 Akanbi, M.A., et al., *Socio-economic factors influencing the utilization of maternal health care services in Amuwo-Odofin local government area of Lagos state, Nigeria*. International Journal of Humanities, Arts, Medicine and Sciences, 2015. **3**(3): p. 1–10.

108 Alam, N., et al., *Inequalities in maternal health care utilization in sub-Saharan African countries: A multiyear and multi-country analysis*. PloS One, 2015. **10**(4).

109 Barros, A.J., et al., *Equity in maternal, newborn, and child health interventions in Countdown to 2015: A retrospective review of survey data from 54 countries*. The Lancet, 2012. **379**(9822): p. 1225–1233.

110 Drummond, P.D., et al., *Barriers to accessing health care services for West African refugee women living in Western Australia*. Health Care for Women International, 2011. **32**(3): p. 206–224.

111 Hamad, R. and D.H. Rehkopf, *Poverty, pregnancy, and birth outcomes: A study of the earned income tax credit*. Paediatric and Perinatal Epidemiology, 2015. **29**(5): p. 444–452.

112 Hodge, A., et al., *Utilisation of health services and geography: Deconstructing regional differences in barriers to facility-based delivery in Nepal.* Maternal and Child Health Journal, 2015. **19**(3): p. 566–577.

113 Gogoi, M., *Association of maternal age and low socio-economic status of women on birth outcome.* International Research Journal of Social Science, 2014. **3**(10): p. 21–27.

114 Solar, O. and A. Irwin, *A conceptual framework for action on the social determinants of health. Social Determinants of Health Discussion Paper 2 (Policy and Practice).* 2010: World Health Organization, Geneva.

115 World Health Organization and UNICEF, *International Conference on Primary Health Care: Alma Ata, USSR, 6–12 September 1978.* 1978: World Health Organization, Geneva.

116 Saturno-Hernández, P.J., et al., *Indicators for monitoring maternal and neonatal quality care: A systematic review.* BMC Pregnancy and Childbirth, 2019. **19**(1): p. 25.

117 Souza, J.P., et al., *The world health organization multi-country survey on maternal and newborn health: Study protocol.* BMC Health Services Research, 2011. **11**(1): p. 286.

118 Shah, A., et al., *Methodological considerations in implementing the WHO global survey for monitoring maternal and perinatal health.* Bulletin of the World Health Organization, 2008. **86**(2): p. 126–131.

119 Souza, J.P., et al., *Moving beyond essential interventions for reduction of maternal mortality (the WHO multi-country survey on maternal and newborn health): A cross-sectional study.* The Lancet, 2013. **381**(9879): p. 1747–1755.

120 Dickson, K.E., et al., *Scaling up quality care for mothers and newborns around the time of birth: An overview of methods and analyses of intervention-specific bottlenecks and solutions.* BMC Pregnancy and Childbirth, 2015. **15**(2): p. 1–11.

121 Lassi, Z.S., et al., *The interconnections between maternal and newborn health – evidence and implications for policy.* The Journal of Maternal, Foetal and Neonatal Medicine, 2013. **26**(1): p. 3–53.

122 Okoroh, E., et al., *United States and territory policies supporting maternal and neonatal transfer: Review of transport and reimbursement.* Journal of Perinatology, 2016. **36**(1): p. 30–34.

123 Malik, M.A., et al., *Expenditure tracking and review of reproductive maternal, newborn and child health policy in Pakistan.* Health Policy and Planning, 2017. **32**(6): p. 781–790.

124 Stenberg, K., et al., *Returns on investment in the continuum of care for reproductive, maternal, newborn, and child health.* 2016: The World Bank, Washington.

125 Arora, N.K., et al., *Setting research priorities for maternal, newborn, child health and nutrition in India by engaging experts from 256 indigenous institutions contributing over 4000 research ideas: A CHNRI exercise by ICMR and INCLEN.* Journal of Global Health, 2017. **7**(1).

126 Lawn, J.E., et al., *Evidence to inform the future for maternal and newborn health.* Best Practice and Research Clinical Obstetrics and Gynaecology, 2016. **36**: p. 169–183. https://doi.org/10.1016/j.bpobgyn.2016.07.004

8 Conclusion

Possibilities for positive childbirth experiences

I started this journey a decade ago in a remote mountain village in Nepal on a quest to find out what needs to be done to save the lives of mothers and babies during childbirth. This is neither the end of the journey nor the final answer to the questions I posed myself in the hope of protecting the lives of many in complex social circumstances who are fighting every day for survival. I feel honoured to be in a position to share with the wider world these stories of loss, struggle and hope told by women living in such a remote location. At the same time, I feel a difficult responsibility in holding the status of researcher while not being able to fully give back to these women who gave of their time, invested trust in me and shared their life stories. Due to the demands of academia and research, I could not give full authority to the stories of the women in my writing, but I strove to present their stories in such a way that the authenticity of their experiences remains alive to readers.

I reflected along the way about the challenges that cross-cultural researchers experience when attempting to simultaneously maintain the research process with respect to the social context of research participants. Balancing research principles with the lived realities of participants is like producing a visually appealing piece of art encompassing deeply embedded stories. I attempted to do this while presenting the lived experiences of these women from remote mountain regions of Nepal. I valued the circumstances of women and argued for taking the socio-cultural environment into account in order to promote childbirth safety and improve maternal, perinatal and newborn survival rates. Rather than creating a dichotomy between a cultural and a medical view of birth, I adopted a collaborative approach which helped to bring to light the context of childbirth and what needs to be done to address issues leading to poor birth outcomes and depressing experiences for women.

Maintaining a critical-feminist and social-constructionist standpoint enabled me to speak to the reality of women. I immersed myself in the everyday lives of women, documenting the stories they shared with me, respecting the way they see themselves and valuing their aspirations for making childbirth a safe, comforting and liberating experience. As women valued their culture, traditions, belief systems, local knowledge, community support, family relationships and social structures in determining safety while giving birth, I supported the view women held of the medical model of childbirth as not being a right fit for them, as it tends to estrange women from their socio-cultural environment. As a result, medically informed policies and strategies in Nepal and other countries of South Asia continue to struggle to address the disparities that remain in maternal and newborn health outcomes. I argued for both policy and practice to acknowledge the broader determinants of health impacting the everyday lives of women, to understand the influence of these determinants on childbirth and to incorporate context-specific strategies to address those determinants which are critical to health and well-being.

It is apparent that childbirth is not merely a biological event or an individual experience for women in a collectivist society. For South Asian women, their childbirth experiences reflect traditions, culture, social expectations and entrenched family values where childbirth is a socially constructed and culturally defined event. In this world view, women do not agree with the intent of medical views which tend to invade the traditions and culture they value the most to ascertain childbirth safety. In cross-cultural communities where women willingly accept social conditions and cultural expectations, attempts to introduce the medical model of care through institutionalisation of women to give birth seem inappropriate. There is no one-size-fits-all approach that can effectively address the factors impacting pregnancy and birth outcomes of women living in complex socio-cultural settings. Remote mountain women provided significant insights into designing context-specific models of childbirth, which offer space for all elements of care required to manage associated risks and to enhance all forms of safety.

The notion of complexity in defining the social circumstances of women in cross-cultural settings was to some extent challenged by these remote mountain women through their view of childbirth as an everyday life event and their sense of comfort in giving birth with the support of trusted women in the community. This made me realise how our language of complexity further marginalise communities as we tend to limit ourselves to what social theories taught us without trying to understand whether the community sees their context in the same way or differently. This example highlights how academics, researchers, policymakers, service planners, practitioners and stakeholders should rethink their use of language, approaches and ways of thinking without assuming complexities about how women see childbirth within their social environment. Women's choices about where and how to give birth must be understood, acknowledged and valued. The decision about childbirth must sit with women, and they should be the ones informing the nature, type and quality of childbirth services that are required in their community.

Researching women in their everyday life settings provides opportunities to learn how constructs of gender, power and relationship influence women and their childbirth experiences. The common use of language to define the status of women: oppressed, disadvantaged, marginalised, vulnerable and underprivileged should no longer be the case. After listening to these remote mountain women in Nepal, I developed a different perspective about structure, agency and power. Knowing how these women living in the remote mountain communities position themselves has provided another important learning. These women did not compare their status with other women living in comparatively resourced environment or find their lives in remote mountains problematic, rather they accepted their circumstances as a given reality and lived with it using the available resources.

For a feminist researcher, this exposure enabled the realisation of how powerful, forgiving and resilient women are in giving comfort to others, as everything these remote mountain women did was for their families. These women did not have any expectations for themselves, and the life they chose to live was to make their children and families happy. As a woman from Nepal, I resonate with these women and their experiences, but I struggle to define my own status as a woman in Western society where I currently reside. Being part of profound conversations and entrenching stories of these women prompted more curiosity of knowing of my own status and the perspectives of others about gender, power, relationship, sense of safety and the meaning of life.

As my main research question was to explore factors that influence the childbirth experiences of women living in remote mountain villages of Nepal, I uncovered many social and cultural factors that intertwined with women's childbirth experiences which were not yet taken into consideration in policy and practice. Women were happy to continue to give birth in a cowshed or surrounding spaces at home rather than making a long and difficult trip to hospital to give birth. There were no childbirth services available to women in the community, and they were asked to come to healthcare centre or the hospital to give birth. It was certainly an unfair call of the health system to those women who cannot deny fulfilling the household responsibilities and committed to follow the social obligations of giving priority to family over their own health, pregnancy or childbirth.

Women frequently challenged the expectations of the healthcare system as being unrealistic and irrelevant to their lives. Many scholars and activists have called such practices a violation of women's rights and demanded access to services for women. With my involvement as an experienced midwife in this research, I understood the challenges that the healthcare system experiences in making services accessible to women and put forward a collaborative solution to address factors impacting women and their childbirth experiences in the remote mountains. I hope the proposed collaborative approach influences policymakers to understand and respond to the socio-cultural needs of women to achieve positive childbirth experiences.

While conducting this research, women's daily struggles of sourcing food to survive struck me the most. Each morning, women are stressed working out what to cook for their family while men are generally occupied with talking about local politics or leaving the village to make money. There is no chance of finding work nearby, as the whole region is experiencing chronic food insecurity and extreme poverty. Culturally, women are the last to eat and finish the day without food if nothing is left in the pot. Even when women are pregnant or breastfeeding, they need to feed other members of the family first. I noticed women working long hours from early morning to late at night to make sure their family did not go hungry. Even after a long day of work, women are still expected to satisfy the desires of their husband, leading to a series of pregnancies which must fit within everyday life routines.

Even though most pregnancies end in the sad reality of loss before or after the birth, women continue childbirth alongside everyday chores to sustain social and cultural expectations. For me, as a midwife and a woman who experienced child-birth in both Nepal and Australia, listening to these stories and sharing them with the outside world through my writing has been both astonishing and challenging experience. While I feel honoured to have been able to collect these stories – I also feel responsible for turning these stories of loss into joyful experiences for younger women in the remote mountains who will soon begin their childbirth journey. As many women shared their hopes for their daughters to live better lives – I feel optimistic that their hopes will contribute to making a difference in childbirth experiences of the next generation women.

It is important that younger women have the opportunity of going to school and making decisions about marriage and pregnancy, so the burden of going through multiple pregnancies and risks of ongoing perinatal losses can be reduced. The current scenario of forcing young girls to get married when they have no option to refuse has led to more critical inequities of maternal, perinatal and newborn health outcomes. Regardless of their socio-economic circumstances, young women must have choice about when and with whom they want to start married life and author-ity to make appropriate reproductive decisions. This will not only contribute to reducing childbirth-related deaths but also help to improve quality of life by pro-viding positive well-being experiences for women.

I was hoping to return to the mountains of Nepal before concluding this book to gain current insights from women about how they view their lives; however, travel became impossible because of the global COVID-19 pandemic. Interna-tional borders are closed and hopes for better days are a long way off as most of us are locked inside our homes for months on end. Nevertheless, during this time I reflected on how women in these disadvantaged communities might have been impacted when they were already struggling to manage everyday life concerns. I could not imagine a happy ending for these remote mountain women at this moment in time, but in the future, I would like to collect stories of women portray-ing happiness and the survival of mothers and babies.

Index

For Product Safety Concerns and Information please contact our EU
representative GPSR@taylorandfrancis.com
Taylor & Francis Verlag GmbH, Kaufingerstraße 24, 80331 München, Germany